Praise for *The Ke*

'*Finally, a holistic approach to health and vitality! Here is a no-nonsense view of the source of illness and dis-ease from the inside out, rather than the outside in. Shann Jones has given us a practical handbook for healthy living based on ancient wisdom and cutting-edge science. I only wish I read this book 20 years ago.*'

PETER MEYERS, CEO STAND & DELIVER GROUP, GLOBAL LEADERSHIP COMMUNICATION

'*I warmly recommend* The Kefir Solution*! Shann Jones has written a motivating and enjoyable book full of useful advice for people with digestive problems and other illnesses. And kefir is magical! I think everybody should introduce it into their lives.*'

DR NATASHA CAMPBELL-MCBRIDE, MD

'*This book provides a comprehensive, easy-to-read overview of the importance of the microbiome and the role it plays in your health. As a reader you'll gain a clear understanding of how your gut goes beyond just digestive issues and can influence your brain, contributing to anxiety and depression. If you've ever wondered how powerful food can be in healing, look no further than the kefir solution – with one drink you'll change the trajectory of your health!*'

DR WILL COLE, LEADING FUNCTIONAL MEDICINE PRACTITIONER AND AUTHOR OF *KETOTARIAN: THE (MOSTLY) PLANT-BASED DIET TO BURN FAT, BOOST YOUR ENERGY, CRUSH YOUR CRAVINGS, AND CALM INFLAMMATION*

The
Kefir
Solution

The Kefir Solution

Natural Healing for IBS, Depression and Anxiety

Shann Nix Jones

HAY HOUSE

Carlsbad, California • New York City
London • Sydney • New Delhi

Published in the United Kingdom by:
Hay House UK Ltd, Astley House, 33 Notting Hill Gate, London W11 3JQ
Tel: +44 (0)20 3675 2450; Fax: +44 (0)20 3675 2451
www.hayhouse.co.uk

Published in the United States of America by:
Hay House Inc., PO Box 5100, Carlsbad, CA 92018-5100
Tel: (1) 760 431 7695 or (800) 654 5126
Fax: (1) 760 431 6948 or (800) 650 5115
www.hayhouse.com

Published in Australia by:
Hay House Australia Ltd, 18/36 Ralph St, Alexandria NSW 2015
Tel: (61) 2 9669 4299; Fax: (61) 2 9669 4144
www.hayhouse.com.au

Published in India by:
Hay House Publishers India, Muskaan Complex, Plot No.3, B-2,
Vasant Kunj, New Delhi 110 070
Tel: (91) 11 4176 1620; Fax: (91) 11 4176 1630
www.hayhouse.co.in

A catalogue record for this book is available from the British Library.

ISBN: 978-1-78817-087-1

Interior illustrations: 1, 45 Andrea Jones and Caitlin Tyler

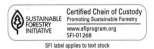

Certified Chain of Custody
SUSTAINABLE Promoting Sustainable Forestry
FORESTRY
INITIATIVE www.sfiprogram.org
SFI-01268

SFI label applies to text stock

This book is dedicated to all the lovely Chuckling Goat clients who were brave enough to tell me their stories. Your honesty inspired me to go looking for answers. You are heroes, all!

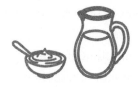

Contents

Author's Note

Kefir is made with living organisms, so every brand of kefir has a unique bio-profile. The results described in the Kefir Solution success stories in this book were achieved using Chuckling Goat Kefir, and I cannot vouch for the actions of any kefir besides our own.

Introduction

You may be wondering if you have Irritable Bowel Syndrome (IBS), or you may be absolutely sure that you do. But one thing is certain:

Tummy's. Not. Happy.

Whether or not you've been diagnosed with IBS, if you experience stomach pain, cramping, bloating, wind, diarrhoea and/or constipation on a regular basis – perhaps accompanied by anxiety or depression – this book is for you.

You're probably feeling pretty overwhelmed at the moment. But here's my promise to you: by the time you reach the end of this book, you'll understand exactly what's going on, and why it's happening. And most important of all: *what you can do about it.*

So, what is IBS?

IBS isn't a disease; rather, it's a wide range of symptoms that occur together. There are no tests for IBS: the history of a patient's symptoms helps a doctor establish a diagnosis.

Until recently, IBS wasn't fully understood, and doctors didn't really know how best to treat it. But the latest scientific research and discoveries have shed new light on this distressing disorder, and its underlying cause is now known. After reading this book, you'll be up-to-date with all the current knowledge in this area.

You'll also have a practical plan that you can put into action in your everyday life: one that has relieved the discomfort experienced by thousands of people just like you.

For a long time, as well as putting up with the distress and embarrassment their symptoms caused, IBS sufferers had to deal with doctors who labelled them as hypochondriacs and told them their problems were 'all in their head'. Nice, right?

Thankfully, these days we're more enlightened, and since around 2010 it's been widely accepted that IBS is a real disorder.[1] IBS is typically diagnosed after a patient has experienced recurrent abdominal pain or discomfort for at least three days per month, in the previous three months, combined with a change in the frequency of their bowel movements or a change in the appearance of their stools.

IBS can occur at any age, but it often begins during the teens or in early adulthood. It's twice as common in women as in men. Studies have shown that people who have a first-degree relative with IBS are at increased risk.[2]

If you have IBS, you're not alone. Simply put, IBS is the most common gastrointestinal disorder in the world. Researchers estimate that up to 15 to 20 per cent of people in the West suffer from it.[3] IBS represents up to 10 per cent of the workload of family doctors and up to 60 per cent of that of gastroenterology practitioners.[4]

According to studies, IBS patients make more visits to their GP, undergo more diagnostic tests, are prescribed more medication, miss more work days, have lower work productivity, are hospitalized more frequently and account for greater overall direct healthcare costs than patients without IBS.

The burden of illness for IBS is significant: research suggests that the disorder can have such a severe impact on Health-Related Quality of Life, that it's been linked to an increase in suicidal behaviour.[5]

If you've been suffering from IBS for a while, you've probably visited your GP and maybe even been referred to a consultant at the hospital. If you were really unlucky, these medical professionals may have suggested you were imagining your symptoms.

If you were 'lucky' and they believed you, you may have been prescribed antibiotics, antispasmodics, laxatives or antidepressants. These medications may have caused troubling side-effects, including nausea, insomnia, palpitations and decreased appetite. And they haven't *really* worked, have they?

So, you may have turned to dear old Auntie Google, and done your own research. Maybe you've cut things from your diet – such as gluten or dairy – in an attempt to cope. Perhaps this helped a little – but it's left you with such a restricted diet that eating isn't much fun anymore. And you're still in pain, still feeling down and are possibly even afraid to leave the house.

But now, finally, there is something that can help. We call it the Kefir Solution. It's all natural, involves no nasty chemicals and its only side-effects are pleasant ones! You may find that while following this natural health programme, you feel calmer, less anxious, less depressed and more energetic.

You may even lose weight, and keep it off. If you have eczema, acne, psoriasis or rosacea, you'll most likely find that it clears up too. Such skin conditions are a common side-effect of tummy problems, and I'll explain why shortly.

In this book, I'm going to share with you some common sense, and some uncommon science, about what's causing your IBS, anxiety and depression – and explain what you can do to feel better. The Kefir Solution has worked for thousands of our Chuckling Goat clients, and it can work for you too!

How I discovered the Kefir Solution

But first, let me tell you my story. I'm not a doctor or a scientist: I'm a farmer's wife and a mother who, when doctors couldn't help us, was forced to search for natural healing solutions for my family. Because of my experiences – none of which I would have chosen! – I know all about feeling frightened, overwhelmed and isolated. And what it's like to struggle with a medical problem for which conventional medicine offers no answers.

I started my adult life in San Francisco as a city girl – a journalist and radio talk-show host – who couldn't boil an egg. I then relocated to Wales, that mythic land of castles, mist and magic. At the age of 41, I fell in love with a Welsh farmer named Rich. We got married and I brought my two children to live with him and his two daughters, on his beautiful farm by the sea.

I was on a steep learning curve as I struggled to adapt to traditional Welsh culture, and started to make my own soap, jam, beer, bread and cheese. In 2010, Rich and I bought our first goat, in order to help my son Benji's bronchial infections (my husband knew of the reputation of goat's milk for easing allergies, asthma and chest infections).

We became enchanted by the goats, and one goat soon became seven. As the herd of goats grew, we needed to use up our surplus milk, so we learned to make a powerful probiotic drink called kefir.

Because we'd met late in life and felt we'd wasted enough time apart, Rich and I started a little business on our farmhouse kitchen table called Chuckling Goat. You can read more about my early adventures on the farm in my book *Secrets from Chuckling Goat: How a Herd of Goats Saved My Family and Created a Business that Became a Natural Health Phenomenon.*

Disaster strikes

When I first met Rich, he'd had ulcerative colitis (a condition that causes inflammation of the large intestine, or colon) for seven years. He was taking some heavy-duty drugs to keep it under control: infliximab and other medications that arrived at our door in a special van, and with their own injector pen.

After a while, these drugs stopped working. During a particularly bad colitis flare-up, Rich checked into hospital and the doctor told him that his large intestine might perforate. He needed emergency surgery.

If I'd known then what I do today about gastrointestinal diseases, I might have had the courage to face down the surgeons and insist that we take a different path to heal Rich's gut. But at that time, I didn't have the knowledge or the confidence to fight that battle. So we began a cycle of surgeries that lasted for four years.

Rich returned home from the second operation *without* his large intestine, but *with* an antibiotic-resistant superbug MRSA infection along the 25cm/10 in surgical incision in his abdomen. It was eating little red holes in the wound that were getting deeper every day – and there was *nothing the doctors could do*.

I'll never forget the day the doctor came to our farm to examine Rich's MRSA infection. The doctor pulled back the long bandage, and the blood drained out of his face. After replacing the bandage, he turned to me and said brusquely: 'I've no experience of dealing with something of this magnitude. I suggest you contact the surgeon who performed the operation.'

Then he packed up his bag, got into his car, slammed the door and locked it, and sped off up our farm track, never to be seen again. I remember grabbing hold of the corner of the table, so my knees wouldn't give out from under me, as I watched him leave.

What were my options now? To whom could I turn? They wouldn't let Rich back into the hospital, because patients were screened for MRSA infection *before* admission. Anyway, how could the surgeon help us? He'd already cut everything out of Rich that could be cut out – there was nothing left. How can you remove an antibiotic-resistant infection that's spreading inside someone's vital organs?

So, was Rich going to be left to die in agony, right there on our sofa, as the infection ate its way into his insides? Well, *that* was just not happening, I determined. Not on my watch. I hadn't travelled halfway across the world, survived so many disasters, kissed so many frogs, fought so hard and finally found the man of my dreams, only to have him die on me three years later. That was *not* the way my happy ending ended.

Bringing it all into balance

So I marched over to my desk, fired up my computer and began to do some research on treatment for MRSA. After a few days, I'd managed to come up with a combination of essential oils that I thought *might* knock back the superbug a bit.

But it wasn't enough. Because while I was researching, I learned that the MRSA infection wasn't just in Rich's wound, and it couldn't simply be killed. *The MRSA had spread all over Rich's body,* replacing every normal skin cell with a copy of itself.

How could I fight all those infecting micro-bugs that were hiding *everywhere* on Rich – in his eyebrows, behind his ears, under his fingernails? Even if I were to dip his entire body in bleach, I could never get them all: some of those bugs would survive to breed and fight another day.

How could I ever kill them all? Answer: *I couldn't. The bad bugs would win, and Rich would die.* Well, I didn't like *that* answer. So I decided to ask a different question.

I'd established that killing all the bugs was a non-starter. In fact, the indiscriminate killing of bacteria was how this whole antibiotic-resistance mess had started in the first place. Medical science had actually created these resistant bugs.

If I couldn't kill all the infecting bugs, then, how could I bring them all into balance? For that, I needed something completely different. I needed *allies* on the microbiotic level that would round up those bad bugs for me. I needed harmony, not death. I needed good bugs to fight the bad bugs and put them back into their box. So where could I find some good bugs?

The answer to that question was sitting right outside: in the stone barn where we made our probiotic goat's milk kefir drink. I knew that the kefir was chock-full of good bugs, and that once they were inside the gut, those good bugs worked to bring the bad bugs back under control. Could it possibly work the same way on the skin, I wondered? Was it even safe to try?

There was no available research to tell me, either way: as far as I could see, no one had ever used kefir on the skin. But with nothing to lose and everything to fight for, I figured I might as well try. By this time Rich was confined to bed, fading in and out of consciousness. The red holes of the MRSA were getting deeper every day, edging closer and closer to his vital organs. So I took a deep breath and set to work.

Back from the brink

Every day for the next fortnight, I washed Rich down with the blend of essential oils I'd created – which I later dubbed CG Oil – alternating with a rinse of the kefir. What I was doing – what I prayed I was doing, anyhow! – was pushing back the bad bugs with the CG Oil, to create a foothold, and then introducing good bugs into the skin biome with the kefir. I was hoping that the good bugs would take over, and wrestle the remaining bad bugs back into balance.

It was crazy. It was stupid. It was preposterous. But it worked!

At the end of the two weeks, Rich swabbed completely clear of MRSA. He got up out of bed, went outside and started up his tractor – and he's been happy and healthy ever since. Today, he runs the farm and physical systems of Chuckling Goat: he designs buildings, manages our herd of goats, keeps me on an even keel, is a wonderful father... and keeps everything else going as well. Thank heavens! My own private miracle.

And I learned something important from this experience:

It's not just about killing the bad bugs that cause disease. It's about adding in good bugs, in order to bring the whole system back into balance.

This is what a probiotic like kefir accomplishes, and it's something that antibiotics can never do. You can't just wipe out bad bugs and leave an empty space, because the bad bugs will creep back in and take it over again. Good health is a space grab. You have to make a preemptive strike with the good bugs – so they take over from the bad bugs. It's all about repopulation.

Once the dust had settled, I sent the CG Oil off to a laboratory, to see if it really had worked, and I wasn't just imagining it. The reports came back, and indeed, the CG Oil was effective against MRSA. It also worked against campylobacter, E. coli and salmonella. Eureka!

Chuckling Goat takes off

Meanwhile, national newspaper reporters started sniffing around, having heard that something extraordinary had happened on our little farm. The press picked up our story, and soon after, the Welsh government sent over an Innovation Sector Specialist to talk to us.

He organized a meeting between Chuckling Goat and the brilliant scientists at Aberystwyth University in West Wales, where our goat's milk kefir was later tested and genetically strained. We've worked closely with Aberystwyth University ever since, and today our Chuckling Goat Kefir is the only university tested and approved kefir in the UK.

Once I'd realized that kefir works on the skin as well as it does inside the gut, I got to work on creating a healing solution for my little boy Benji's ongoing eczema. I discovered that eczema, as well as psoriasis, rosacea and acne, are not really skin problems at all but autoimmune disorders that sit inside the gut. And in order to clear the skin, you must first heal the gut. That's why topical lotions alone will never permanently resolve these conditions.

However, it turned out that drinking kefir *and* applying it to the skin at the same time – in the form of soaps and lotions – *does* work for skin problems! So I learned to put our kefir into Chuckling Goat soaps and lotions. You can read more about the science behind this protocol in my book *The Good Skin Solution: Natural Healing for Eczema, Psoriasis, Rosacea and Acne*.

Reid Tracy, the marvellous President and CEO of Hay House, publisher of my two previous books (as well as the one you're holding in your hands), had faith in our little business. He gave us invaluable advice and invested in us, which enabled Chuckling Goat to grow, and to develop the unique kefir skincare products on which I was working.

As astonished customers found their skin conditions literally clearing before their eyes, Chuckling Goat experienced meteoric sales growth of more than 6,000 per cent in just four years. By 2017, our tiny kitchen table business had grown to 16 employees, 70 goats and 75,000 customers in 26 countries.

Rich's beautiful daughter Elly came to work for us as office manager. Her fiancé Josh joined us as well, and became a brilliant production manager. We found that we loved working closely as a family – and that together, we could deal with pretty much anything that was thrown at us.

Making the connection

But something else amazing was happening, too. Customers who had started taking our kefir to deal with their skin conditions began to report that their *IBS, depression and anxiety had also disappeared.*

THE KEFIR SOLUTION SUCCESS STORY

I've had IBS on and off for a while: I've been through quite a stressful two or three years. My daughter-in-law had terminal cancer and then my husband was diagnosed with cancer, and they died within three weeks of each other.

The stress made my IBS a lot worse at that time. It did make things difficult. Sometimes I'd want to get out early in the mornings, but then I'd have an attack. I'd get pains in my tummy and it would make me a bit dubious about going out until the episode was over.

I tried probiotic capsules and I also went to a health food store and tried things they gave me, including peppermint oil capsules. I don't think they did an awful lot. I went to see my doctor and he said that a good probiotic would help. I saw Chuckling Goat on Facebook, and thought, I'm going to try that.

I began to feel so much better on the kefir, and I'm hoping that the IBS will subside more over time. I'm still grieving, and going through a very difficult time, but I think it's helped with my energy levels. I want to keep on using it until I find I'm not getting the problem at all.

Lots of people like me have tried so many things and nothing seems to help. I just think this could be a great answer for anyone having similar problems. It's a good thing to make people aware of how kefir may be able to help them.

CHRISTINE BRADSHAW, 76, COMPANY ADMINISTRATOR,
HERTFORDSHIRE, UK

Eventually, I could no longer ignore the flood of comments like Christine's and I began to investigate. Once a journalist, always a journalist; I could never resist a tempting question! So... what *was* IBS, and how was it linked to skin issues?

Why was the kefir working for this troublesome condition when nothing else seemed to? What was the connection between IBS, anxiety and depression? Why did all three seem to resolve at the same time when our customers drank our kefir?

Intrigued, I went looking for the science behind these amazing success stories we were seeing – *and I found it.* The result is the book you have in your hands: the Kefir Solution. Now I know it's not just words you're after – you want action! So I've just a few final things to say before we begin.

When you're at the end of your rope

One thing I learned during my journey from city girl to farmer's wife is that life on the farm can be hard. The weather can be brutal. Beloved animals can die. Things can go wrong. Reality is gritty, and sometimes it feels unbearably tough.

So, what to do? Should we become hardened? Should we give in to compassion fatigue, and simply become businesslike about the whole thing?

Hell, no. I decided long ago that the only way around this dilemma was to just *keep right on loving*. Keep my heart open, and keep getting pummelled. Drop my hands away from my face and stop trying to protect myself – just open up to getting whacked, over and over again. Let my heart break, freshly each time, with my full permission.

What does this have to do with you? Well, even though we haven't met yet, I can guess a few things about you. I can guess that your long struggle with IBS, anxiety and depression has broken your heart. I know it feels so unfair that you should have to cope with all this. I'm guessing you feel like giving up. I bet you feel that you're at the end of your rope.

Am I right? But just tie a knot in the end of that rope and hang on. Help is on its way. Be brave. Open to yet another adventure, even if you've tried and failed so many times before. Because when your heart breaks, it's the cracks that let in the light. And we're going to find a way to make those chinks of light bigger and bigger, until the whole problem just dissolves in the light. Stick with me throughout this journey – you'll like what you find at the end!

Now I want you to imagine that you're taking my hand, and that we're going to walk through this together. You're going to be brave, and tough, and honest about what's going on. You're going to take control of this situation, and when our time together is over, you're going to be able to help yourself.

My goal is to give you all the tools you need to resolve your IBS, your anxiety and your depression. You'll have your very own Kefir Solution and it will work for you. How do I know? Because here on the farm, we believe in happy endings – and until you're happy, it's not the end.

Meeting the challenge

Having walked this road alongside Rich, who as I mentioned earlier, had ulcerative colitis for many years before his operation, one of the things I know is that *gut issues are a generally uncomfortable topic of conversation*. My husband is a proud, private man, and I can't count the number of times he bemoaned the nature of his illness.

'Why couldn't it have been my arm, or my leg?' he'd say. 'That would have been so much easier to deal with.'

Well, as they say in Texas, where I was born, *it is what it is*. IBS ain't glamorous, and sure, there *is* a stigma attached to talking about, and dealing with, matters relating to the gut. But squeamishness is a luxury we can't afford here.

So let's take this issue by the scruff of the neck, shake it and look it straight in the eye. No embarrassment, no shyness, and no squeaking around the edges of it, right? Because you can't deal with a challenge until you confront it and call it by its name.

And there's a key word for you as we begin this journey: *challenge*. Dealing with your IBS, depression and anxiety is not an insoluble problem – it's a challenge. Challenges are something to which we rise. Challenges are how we grow.

Meeting challenges is what changes, strengthens and improves us. I've come to the conclusion that being presented with a constant string of challenges, and learning to deal with them effectively, is how the world works. (It's been true in my life, anyhow!)

Challenges are even the way in which your immune system is strengthened. When your body is confronted with a pathogen (a disease-causing microbe), it learns how to cope with it and fight back. Next time round, it's stronger. When you break a bone and it mends, it's stronger in the broken places.

You'll always be presented with challenges – that's a given. The question is: How will you respond to *this* particular challenge? Are you going to give up and sit down by the side of the road? Or are you going to face it with the firm, calm determination to get on top of it, and achieve your own positive solution?

You can't control which challenges you're handed. But *you can control your response.* You'll need to be flexible, determined, disciplined and resourceful, and ready to let go of some old habits, in order to effect your own healing.

I invite you to take the general concepts introduced here in the Kefir Solution and tailor them to yourself. Activate your intuition: put your hand on your heart and listen to what it tells you. You are the only one inside your skin – *you are the expert of your own wellness.* If your instinct tells you to eat or avoid a certain food, then honour that impulse. It will be right for you!

What we're going to discuss here is based on the very latest scientific research from around the world. The ink is still wet on some of this cutting-edge information. It has not yet worked its way through much of Britain's NHS, and your doctor may not even be aware of it. In fact, it may be another 10 years before this ground-breaking knowledge is widely available.

But if you're suffering with IBS, depression and anxiety, I'm guessing you don't have 10 years to wait. So dig in, and share this information with people you know who will benefit from it. We have to help each other along here, until more doctors catch up.

There are, thank goodness, a few brilliant doctors and natural health researchers who are already making full use of the knowledge about the microbiome – they are listed in the 'further reading' section of this book.

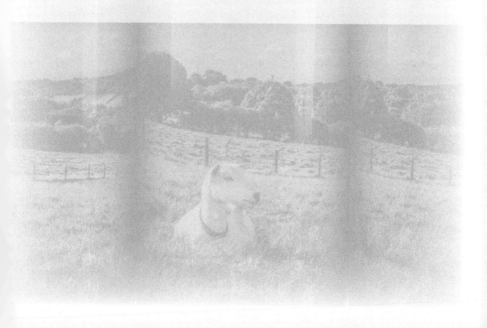

Part One

Uncovering
the Cause
of IBS

Chapter 1

Meet Your Microbiome

As I explained earlier, until very recently, the underlying cause of IBS was not known. But advances in the scientific study of the human gut microbiota – the population of tiny organisms living inside our intestines – have finally led researchers to an answer.

We'll be exploring that answer in depth in the following chapters, but for now it can be summarized as simply as this: if the bugs in your gut get out of balance, you'll get IBS.[1]

Your gut is a natural ecosystem

'What's that?' you ask. 'I have *bugs* in my gut?'

Indeed you do. There are gazillions of microbiota, bacteria, bugs – call them what you will – living inside you right this minute, in something called the microbiome.

The microbiome is the collective name for the enormous colonies of microorganisms, both beneficial and neutral, that coexist with the human body, mainly inside the gut. It's estimated that there are a quadrillion/septillion, or 10^{24}, bacteria inhabiting the gut microbiome. Poetically speaking, that means you have as many bugs in your gut as there are stars in our observable universe.

It may be strange to imagine, but you are really just a walking, talking constellation of different life forms. Essentially, you are the planet, and your gut bugs are the inhabitants. These life forms are all cooperating, competing, fighting, eating and breeding inside your gut, just like in a natural ecosystem.

In fact, they *are* a natural ecosystem, and you're what the scientists call a *holobiont*: a compilation of different kinds of bacteria, plus a host. Like any natural ecosystem, your microbiome is delicate, and it can be easily damaged. What damages it? Modern life! The main things that harm it are antibiotics, stress, sugar and environmental toxins (more on these coming up).

To help you visualize how your inner ecosystem works, and how it can be harmed, let me tell you a story.

PUTTING THE WOLVES BACK INTO YELLOWSTONE

Back in 1872, US government officials decided that the Yellowstone region in Wyoming, Montana and Idaho was an area of such outstanding natural beauty that it should be turned into a national park for everyone to enjoy, forever.

There was only one problem with Yellowstone: there were wolves in the park. And we all know that wolves are bad, right? Nasty, dangerous predators that are the stuff of nightmares and horror movies. So the solution seemed clear: get rid of all the wolves!

The park officials threw open Yellowstone to anyone who wanted to purge the place of wolves. Administrators, hunters and tourists were turned loose with guns, and issued with instructions to round up and kill any wolves they found. And they killed them in huge numbers – by 1926, the last wolf in Yellowstone had been exterminated.

But then something unexpected happened. Without the wolves, the number of elks living in Yellowstone exploded. This booming elk population rapidly overgrazed the willow trees that grew by the rivers' edges. Once the willow disappeared, the beavers that used willow to build their dams began to die out.

Then, because the beavers' dams weren't there to create still, quiet pools in which fish could breed, the fish began to die. Then the birds that ate the fish began to die... so the plants that grew from the seeds carried by the birds began to die. And so the soil microbes that grew on the roots of those plants began to die.

Yellowstone National Park, once famed for its fantastic beauty, began to turn into a desert.

Alarmed, the park's officials started to cull the elk. They did their best, but humans simply don't hunt elk in the same way, and in the same places, that wolves do. The human cull efforts managed to stop the damage from getting worse – but it wasn't able to restore Yellowstone to its previous pristine and biodiverse state.

So in 1995, the authorities took the very controversial decision to put the wolves back into Yellowstone. You can imagine what a fuss that caused! But they managed to do it. The wolves were reintroduced.

And guess what happened? Sure enough, the wolves began to cull the elk. The elk population came down, and the willow trees grew back. The beaver settlements increased from one, back up to nine. The fish came back, and the birds came back, and the plants came back and the very microbes that clung to the roots of the plants returned. Yellowstone bloomed once more.

When your microbiome gets out of balance

Just to be clear here: reintroducing the wolves into Yellowstone ended up altering everything, down to the very *microbes in the soil*, and made the park healthy again. How can this be? It's an example of what scientists call a *trophic cascade*. Trophic means relating to food, and cascade is a series of events that begins at the top and affects things all the way down as it goes, often in complex and unforeseen ways.

Okay, so that's the way nature works, but what does all this have to do with you? Well, *you are a part of nature*. Inside your gut is a natural ecosystem that's as rare, delicate and exquisite in all its biodiversity as Yellowstone National Park.

And just like Yellowstone, your inner ecosystem can get out of balance. For example, if you take antibiotics to kill off the bad bugs in your system, it can have disastrous and unintended consequences – just like killing off the wolves. And without natural predators to keep them in check, the things living in your system, such as candida (a type of yeast), can proliferate and get out of control: just as the elk did in the park.

Now elk aren't bad animals: they're lovely creatures, really. And there's nothing wrong with candida: it lives inside you all the time, and fills a niche in your natural ecosystem. But if the elk and candida are allowed to get out of control – as happens when their natural predators are removed – they can wreak havoc.

What's important is keeping a natural system *in balance*, so that everything can play its part. It's our point-and-shoot mentality – with both guns and antibiotics – that's caused devastation in the natural ecosystems both inside and outside us.

Do you mind? We're dancing in here...

At this point, you may be thinking, *Shann, let's not take this too far. Aren't you stretching the metaphor a bit here, to try to make a point?*

I promise you, I'm not. A recent study undertaken at the Weizmann Institute of Science in Israel revealed that the microbes (bugs) inside your gut are *alive*, and they are literally dancing in there.

They have a routine: like clockwork, they start their day in one part of the lining of the gut, move a few micrometres to the left, maybe the right, and then return to their original position. These small movements can influence a host's circadian rhythms (a 24-hour biological cycle) by exposing gut tissue to different microbes and their metabolites (stuff the bacteria produce) as the day goes by. Disruption of the bugs' dance can affect the host.[2]

This research reveals the gorgeous interconnection between you (the host) and your microbes. You and your bugs are intimately connected; in fact, you interact with them in a permanent, ongoing waltz that cannot be severed.

If your microbes suffer, and their dance falls apart, *you* suffer.

And it's not just the functions directly inside the gut that are affected by the dance of your microbes. They can also affect tissue far away from the gut, such as the liver. Researchers have found that the liver's gene expression changes in tandem with the gut microbiome rhythms. This will impact things like drug metabolism and detoxification, as the liver is the major organ for removing toxins inside the body.

Researchers at the Weizmann Institute seemed awed by their findings: 'What we learned from this study is that there's a very tight interconnectivity between the microbiome and the host,' said the study's co-author, Eran Segal. 'We should think of it now as one supraorganism that can't be separated. We have to fully integrate our thinking with regard to any substance that we consume.'[3]

The four horsemen of the gut apocalypse

Why is this all so critically important to your health? Because the trillions of bacteria dancing inside your gut are essential predictors of success in almost all the systems and levels of the human body: they break down your food and turn it into the building blocks that harvest energy from the diet; they protect against infection; they build skin, bone and muscle cells, and they control hormones, and much more.

The old saying *you are what you eat* **is not actually true. In fact,** *you are what you absorb* **– and what you absorb, is determined by your gut bugs. Wreck the health of your gut, and your overall wellbeing will suffer.**

What wrecks the health of your gut? The main culprits here are what I call the 'four horsemen of the gut apocalypse': diet, antibiotics, stress and environmental toxins such as those commonly found in cleaning solutions and personal care products.

The disruption to the gut microbiome caused by the four horsemen can have countless effects on our health and wellbeing because the damage works its way through our system in a trophic cascade, just like in the Yellowstone story.

But let's focus on how alterations to our gut bacteria affect IBS.

A recent study review found the following:[4]

- **Diet** can alter the makeup of bacteria in the gastrointestinal (GI) tract, potentially contributing to symptoms in patients with IBS.

- **Antibiotic use**, which can disrupt gut microbiota, is associated with IBS.

- **Emotional stress** can change the shape and function of microorganisms in the GI tract.

- **Common antimicrobial agents** can rapidly disrupt gut bacteria.[5]

So, we've established that your health is inextricably linked to the wellbeing of your gut bugs. Damage your bugs, and your health will suffer. And modern life, with its abundance of stress, sugar, antibiotics and environmental toxins, is very hard on your poor microbiome!

THE KEFIR SOLUTION SUCCESS STORY

I was on antibiotics for my skin for three years, and I then took the acne drug Roacutane. I started feeling ill when I was away at boarding school: I suffered from tiredness, and whenever I ate I felt bloated and crampy afterwards. Even worse, for someone my age, was the fact that when I drank alcohol I felt instantly ill.

I tried tinctures, but they didn't work. I had all sorts of tests done, but the doctors couldn't figure out what was wrong with me. I went to a specialist for my tummy, and was given exercises and a very plain diet. I had a colonoscopy, but they didn't find anything.

I went to the doctor and he said to me, 'You have IBS, but there's no solution.' He gave me an antispasmodic drug called Buscopan. It didn't help at all. I preferred the more natural route, and found herbal teas soothing.

My mother has a personal trainer who takes the Chuckling Goat kefir, and one week he over-ordered, so I got some of his to try. The first thing I noticed after starting to take the kefir was that my cravings decreased. Then I noticed I could eat most things. I found I felt full after a meal. And then the pain and bloating disappeared! Even my skin was better when I was taking the kefir.

Then I went away for a week in the summer and didn't take the kefir with me. I noticed a difference by the end of the week: I felt drained again. I started taking the kefir again as soon as I came back, and on the very first day, my tummy sorted itself out. I was so pleased!

I took the kefir from the beginning of summer until mid-October, non-stop, and my issues seemed to be resolved. My parents and I decided that I should do another course of kefir every now and then, just to reset my tummy.

FLORA KILPATRICK, 18, STUDENT, NORFOLK, UK

Chapter 2

The Connection Between Anxiety, Depression and IBS

Scientific research into the gut microbiome has revealed that people with IBS often have anxiety and/or depression – and people with anxiety/depression often end up with IBS.

One of the many studies that show conclusively that IBS, anxiety and depression are connected was carried out in Belgium. In December 2010, there was a massive outbreak of gastroenteritis in two towns in the province of Antwerp, after more than 18,000 residents were exposed to contaminated drinking water.

Obviously, the contamination was a terrible accident, but the team of scientists set up to investigate its long-term effects stumbled across something that they never would have discovered otherwise.

They found that individuals who'd experienced higher levels of anxiety or depression *before* the water contamination developed more severe gastrointestinal infections *after it*. These same poor folk also had an increased risk of developing the long-term complication of IBS, reporting intermittent abdominal cramps, diarrhoea or constipation one year after the contamination.

'Our investigation found that anxiety or depression alters the immune response towards a gastrointestinal infection, which can result in more severe symptoms and the development of chronic irritable bowel syndrome,' reported one of the study's authors.[1]

In other words, anxiety and depression *predispose* the immune system to IBS.

Now, this seems a bit weird, right? I mean, it's easy to see the leap from IBS to depression – IBS is a nasty thing to deal with, and it could make anyone depressed. But this is the other way around: *having anxiety or depression makes you more likely to develop IBS.*

It's also been discovered that childhood trauma or stress make you more likely to suffer from IBS. And the psychological traumas experienced over a lifetime – such as the death of a loved one, a divorce, a natural disaster, a house fire or car accident, physical or mental abuse – have also been shown to contribute to IBS.[2]

Science confirms the role of our gut bacteria

There's also strong evidence that IBS, anxiety and depression are all associated with something called *dysbiosis* (an imbalance inside the gut microbiome) and decreased diversity of the bacterial species in the gut.[3] This what we discussed in the last chapter.

An imbalance of bacteria in the gut has now been definitively connected to IBS. A landmark 2012 study by Cedars-Sinai Medical Center in the USA used cultures from the small intestine to connect bacteria to the cause of the disorder.

Mark Pimentel, an author of the study, said: 'While we found compelling evidence in the past that bacterial overgrowth is a contributing cause of IBS, making this link through bacterial cultures is the gold standard of diagnosis. This clear evidence of the role bacteria play in the condition underscores our clinical trial findings... Bacteria are key contributors to the cause of IBS.'[4]

And that's not all. In 2017, researchers at Canada's McMaster University used faecal transplants to transfer microbiota from IBS patients into germ-free mice, and they found that those mice went on to develop IBS symptoms and anxiety-like behaviour.[5]

It was already known that patients with IBS have certain kinds of bugs in their gut, so the gut bug-IBS connection has been established. But the McMaster study shows that it's possible to start out with the bugs, and use them to create both the gut-related symptoms of IBS *and* the psychological ones – namely anxiety and depression.

In other words, the symptoms don't cause the bugs – the bugs cause the symptoms.

Let's take a closer look at why this is the case.

IBS and the gut–brain axis

It has to do with something called the gut–brain axis, which is the interaction between the brain, the gut, and the bacteria within the gut. New research indicates that in people with IBS, there's a distinct *gut-to-brain pathway*, where gut symptoms begin first, and are often followed by mood disorders.

But there's also a *brain-to-gut pathway*, where psychological symptoms start first, and are frequently followed by gastrointestinal disorders.[6]

The research also shows that if you have IBS, you're 60 per cent more likely to suffer from depression and anxiety than those who do not have the condition.[7] And, as we saw from the experiences of those poor Belgians, it also works the other way around: the brain-to-gut pathway means that if you have anxiety or depression, chances are you'll develop IBS within one year.

Researchers have calculated that in one-third of individuals, a mood disorder precedes a gastrointestinal disorder, but in two-thirds, a gastrointestinal disorder precedes the mood disorder.[8] In other words, your gut issues can be the *cause* or the *result* of anxiety or depression. The brain and the gastrointestinal system are inextricably linked. IBS will lead to depression/anxiety, and those mood disorders will lead to IBS.

It's not 'all in your head'

The gut–brain axis is now so well established that antidepressants are frequently used to treat IBS.[9] Biochemical signalling between the brain and the gastrointestinal (GI) tract can have a major effect on GI disorders.

The normal stress of everyday life can aggravate certain GI conditions. And in a vicious circle – one that you probably understand only too well – worrying about or dwelling on pain, constipation, diarrhoea and other symptoms can make them worse, which in turn increases the stress.[10]

Did you know that you have a 'default network' in your brain? This is basically the way that your brain functions when it's at rest, and nothing much is going on. It processes content with strong self-reference – like when you're thinking about yourself.

Ideally, this default network is suppressed during complex thought processes; we must be able to do this in order to concentrate. But if there's an imbalance of serotonin in our blood, we're unable to suppress this default network – leading to the pattern of poor concentration, negative thoughts and ruminations that we recognize as depression.

Depression really isn't all in your head: it's in your bloodstream and your gut! This means that in the not-too-distant future, doctors will be able to perform a blood test for depression.[11]

IBS and skin problems

In my book *The Good Skin Solution*, I explored the 'allergic march': the connection between hay fever, food allergies, asthma, depression, and eczema. I also demonstrated that IBS is an often overlooked member of that nasty troop.

Science has confirmed that the likelihood of IBS is significantly higher in patients with seasonal allergic rhinitis (2.67 times), those with allergic eczema (3.85 times), and those with depression (2.56 times).[12] So eczema is what they call 'highly correlated to IBS'.

What does that mean for you? It means that your IBS and your skin issues – if you have any – are connected. You may go to the doctor and be told that you have a lot of different problems: IBS *and* depression *and* eczema *and* allergies.

You don't. You have one issue: microbiome damage. All your symptoms are like the leaves of a single tree. And the trunk of the tree sits in your gut. Heal your gut, and these symptoms will all resolve together.

So if you have persistent skin issues, following the Kefir Solution will help sort those out, as well as the IBS, anxiety and depression. Happy endings all round!

IBS and the perception of pain

If you're suffering from IBS, you may feel that you just *hurt* more than other people do. This may be a very small comfort to you, but guess what? You're right!

The human brain can prepare for pain in ways that either increase or decrease the sensation. When expected pain is predictable, tolerable and inescapable, and will result in a reward – say, a doctor's injection to improve our health – most people tell their brain to decrease the intensity of the pain experience. This is a bit like turning down the volume on a speaker, and it makes the body's perception of pain less acute.

But when anticipated pain is perceived as escapable and potentially dangerous – like burning our hand on a hot stove – most of us tell our brain to increase the pain response; this is like whacking the volume on an iPod right up. We can react faster, and minimize possible tissue damage. As always, our brain is trying to protect us.

Now, here's the kicker: scientists have found that IBS sufferers cannot turn down the volume of the pain response – even when expected pain is not dangerous. This makes them more sensitive even to mild discomfort.[13]

Patients with IBS process pain signals from the gut abnormally. And when the IBS is accompanied by depression, it makes everything worse. The more severe the depression, the more pronounced the patients' disturbed brain responses to pain.

What does this mean for you? If you have IBS, chances are that you do not process visceral pain signals generated from internal organs in the same way as healthy people. You're unable to suppress pain signals in the brain and, as a result, experience more pain from the same stimuli.[14]

In fact, the connection between the gut and the brain is so powerful that over time, IBS will actually alter the structure of the brain. Patients who have been suffering from IBS for one year or more show changes to brain grey matter, in areas that relate to attention, emotional regulation, pain inhibition and the processing of visceral information.[15]

Your gut bugs and serotonin

So what's driving the powerful connection between your gut and your brain? It's all down to a neurotransmitter called serotonin, which carries messages inside the brain and gut. You may already be familiar with serotonin's reputation as the 'happy hormone' – one of the key chemicals involved in the regulation of our mood and emotions. Serotonin levels can alter during times of stress, anxiety and depression.

But serotonin does more than just determine how much 'happiness' we are able to experience biochemically. It fills other important functions inside the body, as well. In the gut, among other things, serotonin regulates our bowel routines.[16] In fact, 90 per cent of our body's serotonin is created – and used – in the gut.

From the minute we're born, *having the right amount of serotonin in our system is all about the bugs in our gut.* Scientists have shown that the levels of serotonin we have in our brain as an adult are regulated by the amount of bacteria we had in our gut during our early life.[17]

Alterations to the population of bugs in our gut caused by antibiotics, stress, diet and environmental toxins can have profound knock-on effects on our serotonin levels, and in turn, on our brain/gut function.

Put simply: if something goes wrong with your serotonin levels, you're going to end up with depression and/or anxiety, plus IBS.[18] This is because IBS, depression and anxiety are all tied up with the amount of serotonin inside your system. We'll be exploring the significance of serotonin in more depth in the next chapter.

A new therapy for IBS, anxiety and depression

Connecting the dots between IBS, anxiety/depression and our gut bugs opens the way to finding a solution for this tangle of previously insoluble problems.

The 2017 McMaster University study is a milestone because it moves the gut bug-IBS connection beyond a simple association, and towards evidence that the alterations to our gut microbiota we've been talking about can affect both our gut and our brain.

Most importantly, the study's authors say that their findings 'raise the possibility that microbiota-directed therapies may be beneficial in treating not only intestinal symptoms but also components of the behavioural manifestations of IBS'.[19]

This is the smoking gun that medical science has been waiting for, because it provides the basis for developing treatments for IBS – and its associated anxiety/depression – that are aimed at our microbiota, or gut bugs. In other words: repopulate a patient's microbiome with probiotics and you'll treat their IBS and their depression/anxiety at the same time!

This is really, really good news. It means that we now know the underlying cause of IBS, and how to deal with it. And more good news: we don't need to wait for scientists to develop laboratory-created probiotic therapies to treat IBS because nature has already provided one for us – it's called kefir.

Kefir is a probiotic drink that's made by fermenting kefir culture, or 'grains', in milk. Because kefir contains naturally synergistic combinations of beneficial yeasts and bacteria that are powerful enough to survive the digestive process, it positively affects the diversity and composition of our gut microbiome.

Kefir has been shown to alter the gut in two ways: by adding beneficial species of bacteria and also suppressing pathogens (disease-causing organisms). Kefir has been used for thousands of years, but it's only recently come to the UK, in a slow transit from its starting point in the Caucasus Mountains of Russia. Scientists and doctors here have just begun to explore this probiotic wonder food.

So, what does all this actually mean for you? It means that your gut and your brain are connected, which makes it easier to heal them *together*. By treating your gut and resolving your IBS, the Kefir Solution will also help relieve your anxiety and depression. All three problems *will resolve together*.

Later in the book, we'll explore the power of kefir – and look at exactly how and why it works inside your gut. But for the moment, just relax and understand that there *is* something that has been shown to help both your IBS and your anxiety/depression.

Restore your gut bugs with kefir, and they will begin to produce the right amount of serotonin again. The serotonin will regulate your gut and brain, which will reduce your IBS, anxiety and depression. And your personal ecosystem will bloom again – just like Yellowstone.

THE KEFIR SOLUTION SUCCESS STORY

I suffered from IBS for 10 years, starting in 2008. It began during an awful period of stress at work. As a head teacher, I'd taken on a challenging school, and one particular parent went for me – posting threats on Facebook and so on. It was scary.

Eventually, the police got involved and I had to move house. I also developed severe rosacea, which needed to be covered with makeup every day. I found it upsetting, and the children would ask, 'Miss, what's wrong with your face?'

The IBS was quite severe. I suffered from bloating, and was unable to travel some days. At work, I had to leave meetings in agony, to get to the loo. Even when I hadn't eaten anything, I'd start to sweat and be in extreme pain.

Sometimes I'd be in the supermarket and have to leave my cart, which was embarrassing. I took six months off work, and never went back. When I finally retired, in 2011, I thought I'd come down with flu, but the doctor diagnosed depression.

I started to take kefir in March 2017. I didn't expect a quick fix, but halfway through my first course, I said to my husband: 'Hang on, I haven't had to run to the loo!' After a month, it was amazing. Halfway through my second batch of kefir, I had no IBS and my face returned to a normal colour. I started to feel better and was no longer in pain. I can only attribute the improvements to the kefir – nothing else had changed.

I was also able to come off my antidepressants. You never know if you're depressed or just feeling bad because of the awful episodes: the pain and sweating. You're bound to be happier when that's not happening anymore! In general, I just felt my whole mood lifting. I no longer had that horrible thing hanging over me, thank goodness. I noticed my mood was better in general.

Every six months I think my depression and IBS may be coming back, and I know I need more kefir. I quite like the taste now. I tell everyone I meet who has IBS that they need to get some. I think a lot of people have all sorts of things wrong with them because of modern living and stress.

Since that time, I've moved home twice, and I thought I might have an IBS flare-up because of the stress. But I didn't! All these chemicals aren't doing us any favours. The kefir is magical. It's a natural thing – and that's the way we all need to be going.

PAULINE P., 62, RETIRED HEAD TEACHER, WEST YORKSHIRE, UK

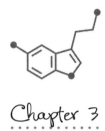

Chapter 3

What's the Big Deal about Serotonin?

As you now know, when you're talking IBS, depression and anxiety, you're talking serotonin. You simply can't avoid it. Since it's so important, let's take a closer look at what serotonin is exactly, and the actions it has inside us.

Serotonin's role in the body

Serotonin plays a role in nearly every bodily process. It regulates your central nervous system, cardiovascular function, digestion, body temperature, endocrinology, and reproduction functions. Serotonin shapes your neurological processes, including sleep, mood, cognition, pain, breathing rate and hunger.[1]

It's responsible for decision-making – even playing a part in social decision-making by keeping in check aggressive social responses or impulsive behaviour.[2]

Serotonin controls peristalsis (the muscular contractions that move food through your body) and is involved in problematic conditions such as vomiting and diarrhoea.[3] Before you were even born, serotonin was involved in your brain, cardiac and pancreas development.[4]

It even turns out that bone growth is controlled not in the skeleton, as was once believed, but in the gut, through serotonin. So for this reason, it makes sense that serotonin levels have been implicated in osteoporosis,[5] as well as rheumatoid arthritis.[6]

People with Alzheimer's disease and severe cognitive decline show severe loss of serotonin neurons, and this loss has now been found to be a major driver of the condition, rather than a byproduct.[7]

Not convinced yet of the importance of serotonin? Let's continue on! Altered serotonin signalling in the skin has been linked to eczema, psoriasis and allergic itch.[8] Low blood levels of serotonin have been linked to self-harming behaviour in teenage girls.[9] A less active brain serotonin system is associated with early hardening of the arteries.[10]

What about when you get 'hangry'? Yep, that's serotonin at work again. Fluctuations in serotonin levels in the brain, which often occur when someone hasn't eaten or is stressed, affect the brain regions that enable us to regulate anger.[11] In fact, serotonin controls our expression of aggression in general.[12]

Levels of serotonin transporters (which remove serotonin) are higher in the brain in winter than in summer, which points to serotonin as the reason why some people experience SAD or Seasonal Affect Disorder, in winter.[13]

Interestingly, there's a difference in the brains of men and women when it comes to serotonin. Depression and anxiety are much more common in women than they are in men. Scientists were puzzled about this – until they discovered that women and men differ in terms of the number of binding sites for serotonin in certain parts of the brain.[14]

Serotonin also appears to control things that are a lot more subtle and difficult to quantify, such as our experience of *meaning* itself. Scientists have found that stimulating one particular serotonin receptor actually created the sensation of personal meaning. This is a potentially significant finding, as depressed patients often report experiencing a lack of meaning in their lives.[15]

Where does serotonin come from?

Sprinkled among the cells that make up the lining of the gut (the epithelium) are some very important ones called enterochromaffin cells, or EC cells for short. There aren't many EC cells – they make up just 1 per cent of the epithelium – but they are the powerhouses of the gut, and have an incredibly important function: they produce 90 per cent of the body's serotonin.

Within the gut lining's villi – beneath the EC cells and other cells – are nerve fibres that sense the movement and contents of the gut, and contribute to intestinal pain and discomfort. Scientists have now discovered that EC cells integrate information about chemical irritants, bacterial compounds and stress hormones in the gut, and then use serotonin to pass that information on to neighbouring nerve cells. From there, electrical impulses travel through the gut's nervous system, and ultimately end up in the brain.

When the EC cells are excited (or 'activated') by certain molecules, they release serotonin into synapses within the nearby nerve fibres. The serotonin triggers electrical impulses in the nerve fibres, moving the signal quickly throughout the gut. The nerve fibres are electrically excitable, and behave in the same way that the brain's motor neurons (nerve cells) behave: passing information and commands that result in movement.

In fact, many of the nerve signals that control your gut come from the gut itself, rather than the brain. The gut is sometimes called 'the second brain' and it helps carry out routine contractions and digestive activities in the gut, without the brain having to get involved.

Scientists now believe that the nerve signals that originate with the EC cells can affect both gut and brain networks, causing involuntary gut contractions. Or, if the signals reach the brain, what could be described as a 'gut ache'.

Just as when you taste something foul and your body tries to get rid of it by gagging, the gut may react to the 'bad taste' of bacteria or irritating molecules by trying to push them out the other end. This could be a way that the gut senses and tries to dispose of bacteria that it perceives as harmful.

Triggering the gut to push out unwanted chemicals and microbes is a normal and healthy mechanism. The problem occurs when the EC cells overreact to normal molecules that shouldn't really cause a problem.[16]

In summary, all of your body's serotonin is produced by a few important cells in your gut called EC cells. Damage those EC cells – with a dose of antibiotics, for example – and your serotonin manufacturing will be seriously impaired.

Your internal communication system

So now that we know what serotonin does, and where it's made inside the body, let's have a look at exactly how it works. Serotonin's function inside your system is all about *communication*.

The brain is a network of around 100 billion nerve cells called neurons, which work by sending signals to one another when they are stimulated. And don't forget your gut – it also contains neurons: 100 million of them! This is more than is found in either the spinal cord or the peripheral nervous system. The neurons in your gut work in exactly the same way as the neurons in your brain.[17]

Neurons communicate with each other by using special signal molecules called 'neurotransmitters'. The 'sending' neuron releases a neurotransmitter, which is bound and registered by receptors at the surface of the 'receiving' neuron. This process triggers a signal, which is sent on to other nerve cells.

After the neurotransmitters have been released between nerve cells, they must be removed to end the signal. This is done by a family of transport proteins that act like little molecular vacuum cleaners in the cell membrane of the nerve cell, where they pump the neurotransmitter back into the nerve cell for later reuse.

Serotonin is one of these neurotransmitters,[18] which is why it affects so many different functions inside the body. It's actually difficult to think of anything important that goes on in your body that serotonin *doesn't* regulate!

However, let's focus now on two important functions of serotonin that affect IBS: the regulation of the mood inside your brain, and controlling the smooth and painless processing of food inside your gut.

We know that gut bugs influence the production of serotonin, because scientists have done the research. A study compared two groups of mice – one containing animals with normal gut microbes and the other with germ-free mice without gut bacteria. It was discovered that the germ-free mice produced around 60 per cent less serotonin than the mice with normal gut bacteria.

And when the scientists restored bacteria colonies in the guts of the germ-free mice, their EC cells began producing normal levels of serotonin again. The study concluded that serotonin levels in the body rely on the interaction between bacteria and host cells.[19]

What's the right amount of serotonin?

Increasing the serotonin levels of depressed patients makes some of them feel better, so for more than 50 years it's been believed that the cause of depression is too little serotonin. The most common antidepressant medications, like Prozac, Zoloft and Celexa, work by preventing brain cells from absorbing serotonin, resulting in an increase in its concentration in the brain.

But these medications are effective in only about *half* of depressed patients, and doctors have never been able to figure out why. However, as we dive deeper into the mysterious world of the microbiome, we're continuing to refine our understanding of how things work in there, and how it affects us.

One of the major breakthroughs has been the understanding that it's the *communication* – or the conversation – between cells that's the important bit. In other words, it's not just the amount of serotonin in the brain that causes the problem: it's a disturbance in the ability of brain cells to communicate with one another.[20]

We now understand that serotonin is an *amplifier*. It has the ability to strengthen the communication between brain cells – like speaking louder to a companion at a noisy cocktail party – making sure that crucial conversations between neurons get heard. In the depressed brain, serotonin appears to be trying hard to amplify that cocktail party conversation, but the message still doesn't get through.

Turns out, it's not about how much serotonin you have. Instead, it's about having a nice even spread of serotonin throughout the brain, so the cross-talk in the brain or gut can continue to relay information without interruption, and the communication can flow smoothly.[21] No one likes being interrupted – not even the neurons in your gut and brain!

Just to drive this point home: serotonin's your internal communication system and it's produced by the EC cells inside your gut. If you wreck your EC cells, your system becomes a chaotic war zone with no proper communications, and no way to carry out the day-to-day business of running your body.

So, here's a quick summary of what we've explored so far:

- IBS, depression and anxiety are all tied up with the smooth functioning of serotonin inside your system.

- Serotonin is the communication molecule that cells use to communicate with each other.

- Poor distribution of serotonin = depression, anxiety and IBS.

Viewing your internal situation through the lens of your new knowledge – and keeping in mind what we've explored about natural systems and the Yellowstone National Park story – I'm hoping that you may think about things a bit differently.

Remember, this is a natural, fragile ecosystem we're talking about here. Imagine if we tried to restore the system itself, to enable it to work more smoothly, rather than just stomping in there with our heavy chemical boots, dumping in random amounts of serotonin with drugs and risking a trophic cascade reaction that we can't anticipate?

Look, your microbiome is a sophisticated and elegant world – one that's based on communication. Your gut bugs are talking, singing and dancing to one another all the time: constantly monitoring the environment, and trading pieces of information to regulate all of the trillions of delicate, complex levels that need to be adjusted in your system at any given moment.

Simply manipulating the serotonin inside your microbiome – up or down – is like taking the wolves out of Yellowstone. Once you've damaged the ecosystem, there will be all sorts of unexpected trophic cascade consequences.

And ultimately, the result for you will be negative. We're just not smart enough to anticipate and prevent all of the potential negative effects. That's why the side-effects leaflet inside any chemical medication packaging is so lengthy and frightening.

The Goldilocks equation

What we need to do is enable the serotonin transmitters to work better, and more accurately, so they can respond perfectly in any given situation. So what we're looking for here when it comes to serotonin is a 'Goldilocks equation'. Millisecond by millisecond, we need the amount of serotonin inside our system to be not too much, and not too little, and evenly spread around. We want the amount to be *just right.*

How do we figure out what's the right amount of serotonin? Well, we don't. There is just no human being on Earth smart enough to do all the instant-to-instant calculations and calibrations that our immensely complex, sophisticated and delicate immune system (our body's defence against infection and illness) can accomplish. Compared to that, our heavy-handed methods of regulating serotonin levels with drugs is pretty brutish and damaging.

How kefir can help

No, we can't solve the problem. *But luckily, nature can.* The technical term for the action we want inside our immune system is 'modulate'. We don't necessarily want to boost serotonin *or* to suppress it: we want the amounts to move up and down, exactly as needed. And what's the best way to do this? By drinking kefir.

Kefir's ability to modulate the immune system is well established.[22] But why does kefir work as nature does? Because it's *natural*: kefir is a living, synergistic combination of bacteria and yeasts – just like your gut microbiome itself.

To keep your gut microbiome in good order, your immune cells, your gut bugs and the cells in your epithelium (gut lining) are working together all the time. If we boost the power of the T cells (the highly specialized defender cells that act as the big bosses of the immune system) in our body, they can do their job better.

The T cells will direct the EC cells inside the gut that make the serotonin,[23] controlling serotonin production like a master conductor with an orchestra. This will sort out the serotonin problems every time, bringing just the perfect mix to each moment.

And what's the best way to boost the action of the T cells inside the immune system? Drinking kefir. Ingestion of kefir has been shown to boost the immune response by stimulating the T cells inside the body.[24] As any good boss knows, it's best to empower the little guys and let them get on with their business. And the same is true inside your body!

Serotonin in a nutshell

So it all makes perfect sense, really:

- Disrupt your gut microbiome with antibiotics, sugar, stress or environmental toxins, and your gut bugs will mess up your serotonin levels.[25]

- The haphazard release of serotonin means anxiety and/or depression in the brain.

- The haphazard release of serotonin also means compromised gut motility, leading to IBS.[26]

- Reverse these processes by taking kefir, and it all gets better – together.

What's tryptophan, and why should you care?

So, we now know that without the right amount of serotonin, it's biochemically impossible for us to experience happiness and wellbeing, or to digest our food properly. But how do you give your body the tools it needs to make the right amount of serotonin?

In order to make serotonin, your body needs L-tryptophan – an essential amino acid (one of the building blocks of protein). Tryptophan is a 'precursor': a key ingredient for making something else. So tryptophan is a precursor for serotonin: without it, no serotonin will be produced. But the body can't make its own tryptophan, so we have to get it from foods that contain it (we'll be exploring these in Chapter 10).

Logically, then, with a decrease in dietary tryptophan you'd expect to see lowered levels of serotonin and increased levels of misery, right? And that's exactly what's been shown in the scientific literature: tryptophan depletion decreases serotonin levels in the brain, which in turn can lead to depression and other problems.[27]

Now let's try it the other way around – when we increase tryptophan, do we see more serotonin and more gut relief? Yes, we do. For example, researchers have found that in mice suffering from intestinal inflammation, increasing the amount of tryptophan in their diet provided relief. The mixture of bacteria in the gut returned to normal, the inflammation died down, and subjects became less susceptible to new attacks.

The connection here, again, is your gut bugs! Studies show that the food we eat can directly alter the mix of bacteria inside the gut, and so influence our health and brain activity.

And more good news – there's hardly any risk of side-effects from increasing our intake of an essential amino acid that's found in our normal diet, like tryptophan,[28] provided we're smart and careful about it.

So, here's a question for you: which readily available medical food contains high levels of tryptophan, as well as offering many other nutritive benefits, and no down sides? Answer: kefir

Aside from being the most powerful probiotic available to us today, kefir also contains tryptophan – in a quick, safe, natural format that will never harm you, that will boost your immune system, ease your gut, lift your mood, raise your energy levels and make you feel better, fast.

So, I'm hoping that you now understand a bit more about what's causing your IBS, anxiety and/or depression. Let's have a closer look at what you can do about it!

Chapter 4

Psychobiotics – Is That Really a *Thing?*

It may be hard to believe that by taking a probiotic like kefir you can alter the composition of your gut bugs in a way that positively affects your mood and brain function, while also resolving your IBS. But as you've just learned, in recent years, a massive wave of research into the gut–brain axis has shown exactly that.

Kefir has been around for millennia, but today it's poised to become a major player in a new frontier in neuroscience because of its actions as a 'psychobiotic'. This is a new term for a combination of live organisms that, when ingested in adequate amounts, produce mental health benefits. In a nutshell, a psychobiotic *is* kefir.

While it's been known for over a century that bacteria can have positive effects on our physical health, it's only in the last 10–15 years that studies have proven there's a connection between the gut, the bacteria in the gut and the brain.

In mice, enhanced immune function, better reactions to stress, and even learning and memory advantages have been attributed to adding the right strain of bacteria to the gut. These bacteria work on the gut–brain axis that we've been discussing.

'Those studies give us confidence that gut bacteria are playing a causal role in very important biological processes, which we can then hope to exploit with psychobiotics,' says Philip Burnet, an associate professor of psychiatry at the UK's University of Oxford.[1]

Psychobiotics have been largely studied in groups of IBS patients, and – drum roll, please – positive results were seen on both their IBS and their depression/anxiety.[2] And there's more good news: you don't need to be clinically depressed to benefit from psychobiotics. The latest research shows that anyone suffering from chronic stress, low mood or anxiety-like symptoms can benefit from them as well.[3]

How do psychobiotics work?

Psychobiotics work on the brain in three different ways:

1. By producing active compounds like serotonin that work on the gut–brain axis. When our gut secretes serotonin, this triggers cells within the gut lining to release molecules that signal brain function and affect behaviour.[4]

2. By working on the body's stress response system, which involves the brain and the adrenal glands.[5] This system, which is also known as the hypothalamic-pituitary-adrenal (HPA) axis, is damaged by chronic stress or illness. When your HPA axis malfunctions, the production of cortisol and other

stress-related hormones goes wrong as well.[6] This plays a big part in causing mood disorders and cognitive problems.

3. By affecting the brain through their anti-inflammatory actions. Chronically elevated levels of inflammation throughout the body and brain, stemming from dysbiosis in the gut, are now known to be one of the major underlying causes of IBS, depression and anxiety. Psychobiotics positively affect the brain by lowering this inflammation.[7]

Psychobiotics can also help boost mood and ease anxiety in people suffering from various chronic diseases. Beneficial bacteria was used in a double-blind, placebo-controlled trial in patients with chronic fatigue syndrome, and the people taking the probiotic had a significant decrease in anxiety symptoms.[8]

In another trial, psychobiotics were shown to help people and animals undergoing stress, by preventing stress-related cortisol increases and raising serotonin levels. Moreover, the probiotic drink that the participants ingested in the trial decreased stress-related physical symptoms such as abdominal pain and cold symptoms.[9]

Psychobiotics and IBS

How about the specific connection with IBS? Psychobiotics have been shown to be a winner here as well. A study found that daily treatment with a psychobiotic for four weeks led to improved mood, reduced anxiety scores and significantly improved quality of life in IBS sufferers.[10]

As for the GI symptoms of IBS, the science showing that psychobiotics work for that side of things is now widely accepted. The American College of Gastroenterology performed a comprehensive literature review on the topic, and found that psychobiotics were both safe and effective in improving symptoms and normalizing bowel movement frequency in patients suffering from constipation or diarrhoea related to IBS.[11]

For reasons that you hopefully now understand, recent science has also shown that psychobiotics may relieve symptoms of depression, as well as IBS. In a study, published in the medical journal *Gastroenterology* in May 2017, researchers found that twice as many adults with IBS reported improvement in coexisting depression when they took a psychobiotic, than adults with IBS who took a placebo.

The study provides further evidence that the microbiota environment in the intestines is in direct communication with the brain.[12]

And lest you think that by choosing a natural solution for your IBS, anxiety or depression you might have to settle for less than the potency of an SSRI (if your doctor has prescribed one), never fear!

One study that compared psychobiotic bacteria to the SSRI Citalopram showed that the bacteria actually worked *better* than the medication in dealing with depression, anxiety and cognitive dysfunction due to chronic stress. It lowered cortisol and restored serotonin and other brain neurochemical levels to normal.[13]

A BRIEF HISTORY OF PSYCHOBIOTICS

The following timeline charts the development of psychobiotics – live, active cultures that benefit brain and gut health – from ancient times to the present day, and documents the interest they have attracted from science and medicine.

8000BCE Origins of the cultured, fermented milk drink kefir: attributed to shepherds in the North Caucasus Mountains in Russia.

7000–6600BCE Earliest evidence of fermented beverages in China, in the Neolithic village of Jiahu.

6000BCE Origins of yogurt: attributed to Neolithic peoples of Central Asia.

3700BCE First appearance of kumis, a fermented milk beverage made from mare's milk: attributed to the nomadic people of Central Asia.

300BCE–CE200 Emergence of nattō, a food made from fermented soya beans, in Japan.

200BCE Origins of sauerkraut: attributed to the Mongols in the north of China, then later introduced to Europe by migrating tribes.

1600s The 'Father of Microbiology', Antonie van Leeuwenhoek, is the first to observe microorganisms under a microscope.

1857 In France, chemist Louis Pasteur proves conclusively that fermentation is initiated by living organisms.

1907 Introduction of the concept of a 'probiotic': this is generally attributed to the Russian-born Nobel Prize co-recipient Élie Metchnikoff, who suggested the possibility of colonizing the gut with beneficial flora.

2006 The first study on the human microbiome is published in the journal *Science*.

2008 The United States National Institutes of Health (NIH) sponsors the Human Microbiome Project, with a goal of testing how changes in the human microbiome are associated with human health or disease.

2012 Founding of uBiome: a biotechnology company taking a citizen science approach to sequencing the microbiome. The American Gut project is launched: the world's largest crowdfunded citizen science project.

2013 Timothy G. Dinan, Catherine Stanton and John F. Cryan, from the Alimentary Pharmabiotic Centre in Ireland, define a 'psychobiotic' as a living organism that, on sufficient ingestion, produces a health benefit in patients with psychiatric, or neurological, illnesses.

April 2014 Chuckling Goat Ltd begins to produce traditionally made kefir with real grains on a large scale in the UK. Thousands of clients report that their IBS, depression and anxiety symptoms are ameliorated by the kefir.

July 2016 A systematic review of 15 human randomized, controlled trials finds that certain commercially available strains of probiotic bacteria possess treatment efficacy (i.e. improved behavioural outcomes) in certain central nervous system disorders – including anxiety, depression, autism spectrum disorder, and obsessive compulsive disorder (OCD) – and improve certain aspects of memory.

October 2016 Dr Diego Curro, lead author of the *British Journal of Pharmacology*, publishes a comprehensive literature review stating that probiotics appear to be effective in ameliorating IBS symptoms.

January 2017 The BBC television series *Trust Me, I'm a Doctor* shows that traditionally made milk kefir produces the most statistically significant effect inside the gut of any probiotic food.

So cutting edge, even the military is interested

Is all this stuff about psychobiotics just a bunch of scientists doing on-the-edge research? Certainly not – the US military is investigating it as well! The US Office of Naval Research is sponsoring research into intestinal bacteria and their effect on the human brain and mood.

'This is extremely important work for US warfighters because it suggests that gut microbes play a strong role in the body's response to stressful situations, as well as in those who might be susceptible to conditions like PTSD,' says Dr Linda Chrisey, a programme officer in ONR's Warfighter Performance Department.

ONR is supporting research that's anticipated to increase warfighters' mental and physical resilience in situations involving dietary changes, sleep loss or disrupted circadian rhythms from shifting time zones or living in submarines. The research so far shows definitively that treating gut bacteria can seriously affect mood and demeanour, improving stress behaviours dramatically and with lasting results over time.[14]

The science is in! Psychobiotics like kefir work for IBS, depression and anxiety. There are no nasty side-effects and a multitude of positive effects, which may include weight loss and improvement in a number of other body functions.

THE KEFIR SOLUTION SUCCESS STORY

My mother's been unwell for a while: she has dementia and a history of IBS. Her IBS was really bad, and she had all the hospital checks, camera tests, special diets, etc. But they couldn't find anything wrong, and couldn't give us anything that helped.

Then I heard Shann Nix Jones on the radio, talking about kefir. Afterwards, I took the plunge and ordered some. I was sure my mother would reject it, as she has a phobia of milk, but she drank it! She says it tastes like buttermilk, and that it reminds her of the old farming days.

The kefir has made the biggest difference to my mother's health: it's just completely reversed the IBS. Before, she was avoiding most foods, so she was underweight, and she had to take antacids after every meal. But that's all stopped. I can sneak eggs into her diet now: I whisk them up with cheese and put them on toast. I couldn't have got her to eat that before, as she would have been ill afterwards. Her wellbeing has improved, she's eating more and for the first time in a long while, she doesn't have heartburn.

She has a vascular condition, and her legs were always discoloured. But not long after she started drinking the kefir, I noticed that her legs were a normal colour. She also has asthma; but we went down to one inhaler, and now we're on no inhalers!

Kefir is insurance for things going wrong. But you can't just take it on its own: you have to do it hand-in-hand with the entire Kefir Solution, in particular reducing sugar. The programme has been a major factor in reducing my mother's stress levels, and she also gets a better night's sleep now. She used to nap all the time, but she's stopped doing it during the day. I also take kefir, and have noticed the difference in my stress levels and panic attacks.

My mother's stomach is so much better than it was. Now at her consultations, no one talks about IBS. That has been a massive difference: I wouldn't want to find out how she'd be without it.

TAMMY SHAIKH, 47, KENT, UK, A CARER FOR HER 75-YEAR-OLD MOTHER

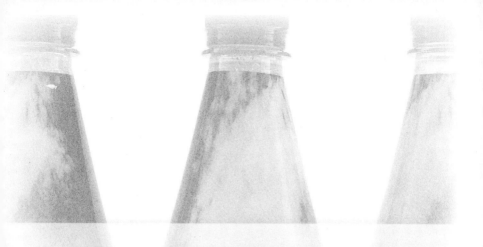

Part Two

The Kefir Solution: A Five-Step Healing Programme

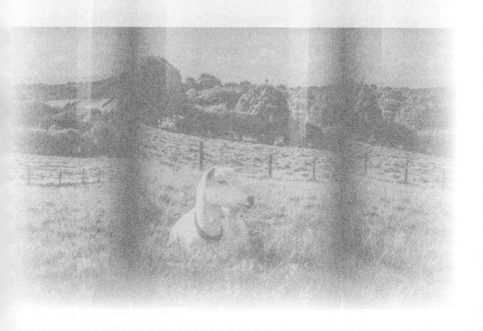

Chapter 5

Introducing the Kefir Solution

As you now know, kefir is a powerful natural remedy that puts good bugs into your gut to aid your microbiome, *and* adds dietary tryptophan to your system to enable you to produce more serotonin, which will boost your mood and enable smoother digestion.

But here on the farm we've discovered over time that as well as drinking kefir, there are *other* actions we can take to support and boost the effect of the probiotics inside our system. Together, these actions create a powerful virtuous healing spiral inside the gut that we call the Kefir Solution.

How to follow the programme

There are five steps to the Kefir Solution. In the following chapters, you'll discover the cutting-edge research behind each step, and learn how following the programme can help heal your IBS, anxiety and depression – all at once.

1. **Step #1:** Drink kefir

2. **Step #2:** Take ashwagandha

3. **Step #3:** Lean in to your feelings

4. **Step #4:** Alter your eating habits

5. **Step #5:** Make lifestyle shifts

So first you're going to drink kefir – which will reset your gut microbiome – and then you're going to pursue certain principles around food, your feelings and lifestyle that will support that change. It's a bit like farming. You have to plant the seeds, and then you have to tend to their growth. Both parts of the equation are equally important.

Will the kefir work on its own? Well, it won't if you're putting certain other things in your gut at the same time. Like antibiotics, for example: as I said earlier, that's like putting fish into a river and then pouring bleach in. The same thing applies to sugar, which kills off your good gut bugs and feeds your bad gut bugs. So drinking kefir while eating sugar is a waste of time.

The Kefir Solution FAQs

Two questions often come up when people ask me about following the Kefir Solution: *How long do I have to drink the kefir?* and *How long do I have to follow these eating and lifestyle principles?*

Personally, I drink kefir every single day of my life, and I plan to do so forever! My microbiome (and yours, and everyone else's on this planet!) is under constant assault from prescribed antibiotics (and those in the food chain), pollution, environmental toxins and stress.

This means that those precious little gut bugs are being attacked every day. Why wouldn't I take constant protective measures to shore up my microbiome and boost the activity of the hardworking immune system warriors in there?

But the short answer is: take the kefir daily until you see the health results that you want. That would be when your IBS disappears, your mood lifts, your anxiety disappears and your skin is clear. At that point, you can ease off and take one 21-day 'course' of kefir every three months. I think of these as seasonal immune boosters.

If your symptoms reappear, you'll know that you've backed off the kefir too soon. Begin taking it again, until your symptoms disappear once more. In this way you become the expert of your own wellness – you can just use the kefir as needed, until you feel better.

The same goes for the eating principles in this section. What I'm suggesting here is not a fad diet, but a long-term, slow and steady shift in your overall behaviour patterns. Along with the lifestyle changes, these eating principles will reduce inflammation inside your system, increase joy in your life and support every system in your body.

On the farm, we eat (and act) in this way every day. After years of following the Kefir Solution we're all free from any major skin, gut, health or mental health issues. We work hard and play hard. It's been longer than I can remember since any of us had a streaming head cold or had to take a course of antibiotics. The principles of the Kefir Solution have become habitual for us.

At this point I should say that we do follow the 80-20 regime – we're good for 80 per cent of the time and have treats for 20 per cent of the time. For example, I consider bread to be a treat. I love it, and have it on special occasions, but I don't eat it every day.

Track your progress

As you work with your IBS, anxiety and depression, give yourself a nine-week window during which you plan to be exceedingly strict about following the Kefir Solution. Keep track of everything you eat, be sure to take the kefir every day and follow each step of the programme to the letter.

Monitor your progress in a journal, in which you write down every symptom that you have and give yourself a numeric marker, 1–10, for how that symptom is each day.

Be patient

Be aware that natural healing is slow and takes time! We've become accustomed to taking chemicals that instantly cover up our symptoms, but leave the root of the problem intact. The Kefir Solution is a different process – you're reseeding your microbiome with the good little plants it needs to heal. In doing so, you'll actually be resolving the problem, not just temporarily suppressing it. Your results will be real, *but gradual.*

Imagine that you've asked me for an apple, and in response I've handed you an apple *seed*. You're going to have to plant that apple seed, water it, nourish it and wait for it to grow. It has to develop into a sprout, a sapling... and then set flowers that develop into fruit. It's going to take a looong time!

That apple, when it's ready, is going to change your life. But you're going to have to cultivate patience, and interact with the whole natural healing/growing process! And patience is a habit that we have lost.

So dust off your genetic natural healing habits. Deep in your DNA, there are generations of people who used natural healing, and understood the power of restoring the system and giving it time to work. We've used these natural healing remedies for far longer than we have the chemical ones – and all that knowledge is still there in your cells. Let it out!

THE KEFIR SOLUTION SUCCESS STORY

As a child, my son was constantly on antibiotics for ear infections and chest infections. He was diagnosed with chronic constipation, along with visceral hyperalgesia (the experience of pain within the inner organs, or viscera, at a level that is more intense than normal).

Recently, he was off school for 18 months and home-schooled, because he was on so much medication and in so much pain. In November, he said, 'What's the point in living? If this is life, there's absolutely no point.' I was constantly calling up the consultant, saying: 'This is ridiculous, and you have to do something! All the medicines you're giving him must be stripping all the goodness out of him, and putting nothing good back in.'

It got to the point where his body was jumping like he was having electric shocks, and he was dripping with sweat because he was in so much pain. This seemed to have come from nowhere, and it had such a bad grip on him, it was unbelievable. His tutor came to see us, and said, 'Have you heard about Chuckling Goat?' so we ordered some of their kefir.

Within the first day of using it, my son's condition turned around. He said, 'I feel a bit better.' The next day he woke up and said, 'I don't think I've got pain anymore.' A couple of days after that, he still didn't have any pain. When you've been in pain for so long, it's almost hard to believe.

I also found it hard to believe that he could be feeling better within days of starting on the kefir, so I called Chuckling Goat and asked, 'Is it normal for it to happen this quickly?'

We saw our consultant two weeks after starting the kefir and he said, 'I don't know whether this is a placebo, but if it's working, that's great. We'll see you again in six weeks, together with another consultant, and see how things are then.'

When we returned six weeks later, things had gone from strength to strength and the consultants were amazed. I'd already started reducing the tablets and it was agreed we'd keep reducing them to see the outcome. My GP said it was amazing: what a transformation. I kept him on the kefir for 12 weeks. We haven't been back in touch with the consultant since, and no longer take any medication.

My son is a big believer in the kefir and whenever he feels his stomach flaring up, or if he's about to embark on a difficult period, he will order some to help him through. It has made a massive difference to his life.

Go and get kefir. This has totally turned him around. Coincidence? I don't think so. I'm absolutely 100 per cent convinced: what else could it be? If it's working for you, you know it. It's absolutely brilliant and I would recommend it – it was our life-saver.

A.J., CEREDIGION, WALES. HER 16-YEAR-OLD SON WAS SUFFERING WITH INTENSE IBS

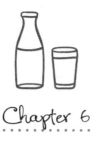

Chapter 6

The Kefir Solution
Step #1: Drink Kefir

So we've examined the science behind what kefir is and how
it works, and now we're ready to get started on the Kefir
Solution. The first step, logically enough, is to drink kefir!

If you hadn't heard of kefir before picking up this book, don't
worry – you're not alone. This potent probiotic drink, made by
fermenting milk with a living kefir culture ('grains') that contains
multiple strains of beneficial bacteria, is a relative newcomer to
the probiotics market in the UK, although it's much better known
in Russia, Eastern Europe, the USA and Ireland.

You can buy ready-to-drink kefir, or you can source your own
kefir grains and follow the instructions that come with them. But
why should you choose to take kefir rather than one of the many
other probiotic foods, drinks and supplements out there?

In recent years, scientific research, and subsequent media
interest, in the gut microbiome has exploded. Food and drink

manufacturers have responded to this by creating a multitude of probiotic products, including kefir, that claim to improve our gut health and our overall wellbeing. But a question remained unanswered: *Do any of them actually work?*

Putting kefir to the test

In January 2017, the first mainstream UK study was performed to determine which of these probiotics has the greatest impact on the bugs inside the human gut. Dr Michael Mosley, presenter of the BBC TV show *Trust Me, I'm a Doctor*, set up a trial in Inverness, Scotland, with the help of NHS Highland, and 30 volunteers and scientists around the country.[1]

The volunteers were split into three groups and over four weeks each one was asked to try a different probiotic food or diet. The first group tried an off-the-shelf probiotic yogurt drink of the type found in most supermarkets and shops. The second group tried kefir. And the third group was asked to eat foods rich in a *prebiotic* fibre called inulin, which is found in Jerusalem artichokes, chicory root, onions, garlic and leeks. (The easiest way to understand prebiotics is to think of them as 'food' for the good bugs, or probiotics.)

At the end of study period, the biggest change in gut bacteria was seen in the group that had taken the kefir. This confirms that the non-transient bacteria in kefir *do* survive our digestive process – with its strong acid that kills off dangerous bacteria in our food – and reaches the gut to colonize it and suppress disease-causing bugs.

'Fermented foods [like kefir] by their very nature are quite acidic and so these microbes have had to evolve in order to cope with these sorts of environments. So they're naturally able to survive in acid,' says Dr Paul Cotter from the Teagasc Research Centre in Cork, who helped with the BBC study's analysis. 'That helps them to get through the stomach in order to then have an influence in the intestine below.'[2]

Is all kefir created equal?

Once the BBC experiment had established that kefir is indeed effective inside the gut, the next question was, *does it matter how the kefir is made?* After testing a selection of shop-bought and traditionally made (homemade-style) fermented products in a laboratory, the *Trust Me I'm a Doctor* team found some remarkable differences between them. While those made by traditional methods contained a wide range of beneficial bacteria, some of the commercial products contained hardly any.

The researchers determined that many of the commercial probiotics available from the supermarket, including kefir, are typically subjected to pasteurization *after* preparation, to ensure their safety and extend their shelf life. The problem with this is that pasteurization kills off all the bugs, both good and bad, so those products have very little impact on the gut.

Note: I need to clarify that it's okay to *begin* the kefir-making process with pasteurized milk; in fact, as we'll discuss later on, you can use many different kinds of milk to make kefir. The bacteria in the kefir will always trump the bacteria in the base, meaning the kefir grains will populate the milk base with their own strains of bacteria, whether the milk is pasteurized or not. But if you pasteurize the *finished* kefir, you've undone all your hard work by killing off all the good bugs you've carefully put in there.

So, only homemade or traditionally made kefir, made with real grains and with the final drink left unpasteurized, will produce the powerful gut-healing effect you're after.[3]

Milk kefir versus water kefir

There are two different kinds of kefir: water kefir and milk kefir. Water kefir is made with water kefir grains, and milk kefir is made with milk kefir grains. The difference between the two is that milk kefir is far more powerful than water kefir. For the Kefir Solution, my recommended daily dosage for milk kefir is 170ml/6fl oz, but if you're drinking water kefir, you're going to have to drink at least 560ml/1 pint per day.

Why is this? According to the American Society for Microbiology, it's because probiotics' success in boosting human health depends partly on the food, beverage or material that's carrying them, and dairy provides the strongest base for probiotics.[4]

Another reason that milk kefir is superior to water kefir is that it contains lactoferrin, an important iron-binding protein that has many functions in the immune system, including offering protection from bacterial, viral, fungal and protozoal infections. Lactoferrin is so powerful and multifunctional that it's been described as the 'Swiss army knife' of the human host defence system.[5]

At Chuckling Goat we tried making coconut water kefir for a while, but discontinued it after we found that it just didn't produce the powerful 'wow' results we were after for our clients. I'm also not a fan of adding refined sugar to things, because of the damage it causes in the microbiome; and to make water kefir, you need to add sugar to the mix, for the grains to eat.

If, however, you're vegan or specifically allergic to goat's milk, any kefir is better than no kefir as a way to get those good bugs back into the gut – so you should investigate coconut water kefir. If you make coconut water kefir at home, be sure to ferment it until *all* the added sugar has been consumed.

Please note also that most people who believe they are allergic to all dairy are generally only allergic to cow's milk, which contains a very common allergen called A1 casein. Goat's milk is considered to be a hypoallergenic food, which is why it's used in baby formula all over the world. Many babies are able to tolerate goat's milk even when they are allergic to their own mother's milk. It's possible, although very rare, to be allergic to goat's milk. This is a matter for an allergy test to determine.

Which type of milk is best for kefir?

So, we know that dairy is the most powerful base for probiotics, and that milk kefir is your best choice, if possible. Note that if you choose to make your own kefir, it's important to use full-fat (whole) milk, as the milk actually feeds the kefir grains, and they need a full spectrum of fats and minerals to survive.

But milk kefir made with which kind of milk? According to Dr Josh Axe, a clinical nutritionist and doctor of natural medicine, goat's milk outperforms cow's milk in the following ways:[6]

1. Goat's milk is easier to digest than cow's milk.

2. It has fewer allergenic proteins and causes less inflammation.

3. It's high in calcium and fatty acids but low in cholesterol.

4. It's beneficial for the skin.

5. It absorbs nutrients and minerals better than cow's milk.

The scientists agree: researchers in Granada, Spain, who were studying the relative benefits of goat's and cow's milk, found that goat's milk was more beneficial to human health. They found reason to believe that goat's milk can help prevent conditions such as anaemia and bone demineralization. Goat's milk was also found to help with the digestive and metabolic utilization of minerals such as iron, calcium, phosphorus and magnesium.[7]

People also often ask about kefir made with other types of milk – such as coconut milk, rice milk, nut milks, oat milk and soya milk. I don't recommend coconut milk kefir, as it's a processed food that frequently contains guar gum (which can cause digestive issues); it's also been identified as a FODMAP (a short-chain carbohydrate that can contribute to gastrointestinal disorders): two good reasons why people with IBS should avoid it.[8]

I'm also not a fan of soya milk. It's an endocrine interrupter and contains high levels of phytic acid, which impairs the absorption of iron, zinc and calcium, and may promote mineral deficiencies.[9]

Nut milks, oat milk and rice milk are okay for IBS sufferers – oat milk is particularly good, as it's anti-inflammatory and calming to the digestive system. These milks may be used as a base for milk kefir, but milk kefir grains will not survive in them over time: you'll need to rotate your grains back into animal milk on a regular basis to enable them to survive.

What about powdered probiotics?

Some of our clients have previously tried other kinds of probiotics: powdered and desiccated varieties, for example. They ask me if they should continue taking these dried probiotics once they start drinking goat's milk kefir on the Kefir Solution.

The answer is a simple 'no'. Kefir is exponentially more powerful than these dried probiotics, and it renders them completely irrelevant for a number of reasons:

1. Dried probiotics generally contain just one or two strains of bacteria, compared to kefir's natural synergistic mix of multiple strains. This is like comparing one or two birds to a whole jungle of them.

2. Dried probiotics are desiccated and on their way towards death, which is why the number of bacteria in them will decrease over time. Kefir bacteria are living and thriving in their own environment, increasing in number all the time and becoming more powerful as they go.

3. Probiotics need a food source, which is called a prebiotic. If you take probiotics that have been artificially extracted, you also need to provide them with the proper food source, or they won't work. This can be complex. Kefir is what's known as 'synbiotic': it contains its own food source in one neat natural package – prebiotics and probiotics together. So the bacteria already have everything they need to thrive.

GUIDELINES FOR MAKING YOUR OWN KEFIR

Working with live cultures can be a wonderful boon to health. It's easy to make your own kefir at home: kefir grains can be ordered online. Like anything, however, homemade kefir has both benefits and potential risks – and often the risks are not described in the instructions that accompany the grains.

So, in order to ensure that your homemade kefir is safe for consumption, please observe the following food safety guidelines:

✤ Ferment your kefir until the pH is below 4.5. This is the level at which most bacterial pathogens are unable to survive. pH meters are widely available for this purpose. Drop the pH of your kefir down to 4.5 or below as rapidly as possible.

Although it's fine for the entire fermentation process to take up to 48 hours, this initial drop in pH needs to happen quite quickly – ideally within the first 16 hours of fermentation. Otherwise you run the risk of spoilage bacteria entering your kefir.

✤ The ideal ratio of grains to milk is about 1:7. Fermentation rates vary, depending on heat and activity (both of which increase fermentation rates), so keeping your kefir warm and shaking it from time to time will speed up the fermentation process.

✤ Test your finished kefir at a public health laboratory *on a regular basis*, to ensure your grains have not become contaminated. Whenever you reuse a live culture (such as kefir grains), you run the risk of bacteriophage contamination.

Bacteriophages, or 'phages' as they are known, are viruses that infect bacteria. They are found in ecosystems where bacteria are commonly found, including man-made ecological niches such as food fermentation vats or jars.

Bacteriophages can turn harmless bacteria into agents of disease, by transferring to them genes that produce toxic substances.[10] These bacteria are then able to infect humans and cause food poisoning and other potentially deadly diseases.[11]

At Chuckling Goat we have our kefir regularly tested by a microbiology lab to ensure that it's free from any phage or pathogen infection. I strongly recommend that if you're making kefir at home, you do the same! Otherwise you run the risk of a phage infection getting into your grains, which if you continue to use them, will propagate the phage contamination.

As it's not possible to sterilize the grains themselves, this is quite a risk for the home producer who does not test their kefir for purity. If you contact the public health laboratory nearest to you, they can explain how you can bring in your kefir for testing. Ask for a standard microbiolocal food safety screen, for a live culture product. (They may never have heard of kefir!)

How to take your kefir

Kefir is strong stuff, so I recommend you start slowly. Take one tablespoon of kefir per day, and as your system adjusts, work your way up gradually to a daily dose of 170ml/6fl oz. Choose pure goat's milk kefir that's been made with real kefir grains, and has no added sugar, sweeteners or flavourings. Drink it first thing in the morning, on an empty stomach.

Why on an empty stomach? Because tryptophan only works on the brain when consumed on an empty stomach.[12] Why first thing in the morning? Because the lactate in kefir (not lactose: kefir is 100 per cent lactose-free) will give you an energy boost, and you don't want that last thing at night or you'll have trouble getting to sleep.

Is it okay to drink liquids before drinking the kefir? Yes, but give them 15 minutes or so to clear your system before you take your kefir. The idea here is to give the live bacteria in the kefir a nice clear run at the wall of the gut, to which they'll adhere and begin fighting for space with the bad bugs that are parked there, and start pushing them out.

How soon can you eat after drinking the kefir? Just give the kefir bacteria about 15 minutes to get settled in, and then go ahead and eat. It's okay to use your daily dose of kefir to make my overnight kefir oats breakfast (*see recipe on page 146*), or add it to a smoothie, but take the kefir *before* eating a large, greasy meal that would coat your intestines and block the kefir's absorption.

You can sweeten your kefir by adding 100 per cent pure stevia (see Chapter 10: The Kefir Solution Eating Principles) or blend it up with fruit, but if you do the latter, be sure to consume it *immediately*. Don't let it sit overnight, as the fructose (fruit sugar) will degrade the power of the probiotics.

Dealing with detox symptoms

Depending on the level of your dysbiosis – how severe and longstanding your IBS, depression and anxiety are – you may experience a detox while you're taking the kefir. This is because the good bugs are going in to do their spring-cleaning work inside your system, and pushing the bad bugs out. Detox symptoms may include headache, nausea, dizziness, diarrhoea or constipation, or a flare-up of a skin condition.

These are temporary side-effects and they will pass. *Do not stop taking kefir in the middle of a detox!* These symptoms are a sign that your microbiome needs help, so don't leave it stranded.

If your detox symptoms become too intense, reduce your daily dose of kefir to one tablespoon until things settle down, then increase the amount again gradually. Your hands are on the controls here: increase or decrease as needed, until you're at your own cutting edge of improvement, without too much discomfort.

Is it possible to overconsume kefir? Well, the Russians drink 560ml/1 pint of it a day. I've had Russian customers tell me that our 21-day course would only last them a week! Again, you're the expert of your own wellness here – experiment to find the daily dose that's right for you.

THE KEFIR SOLUTION SUCCESS STORY

I've had IBS for about 13 years: it started with the stress I experienced when my father passed away. I wasn't able to eat bread or pasta because my stomach would become really bloated. I experienced anxiety and depression as well: I was very upset and low.

The anxiety meant that I worried about everybody and everything, all the time. I really worried about my family. It was a very sudden knock-on effect. I started having panic attacks.

I tried all the different tablets for IBS that the doctor gave me – Buscopan and peppermint oil, etc – but they didn't work. I was about to give up when I saw Chuckling Goat featured on the TV show Back to the Land. *I tried some of their kefir and lo and behold, it worked!*

On the first course, I became less uncomfortable. By the middle of the second course, the IBS had gone. I took a third course, and it didn't come back. I took four courses altogether, and the IBS is now cured. It's brilliant.

I certainly noticed a difference in my mood and energy level. I felt a lot better. My mother always laughed at the face I made when I took the kefir, but it definitely lifted my mood when I was having it. I'm not having panic attacks anymore.

I would 100 per cent recommend kefir. I was amazed – I had no stomach bloating, no cramps: just complete comfort and a normal tummy! Fantastic! I'm so grateful for my new lease of life!

CAROLINE DEBNAM BARBER, 36, HERTFORDSHIRE, UK

Chapter 7

The Kefir Solution Step #2: Take Ashwagandha

So, the kefir will get to work on putting those good bugs back into your gut. But natural healing is a slow process, and in the meantime, I'm guessing that you need an immediate boost: something that will relieve your stress, ease your anxiety and depression, and even enable you to get a better night's sleep. Right?

I'm going to suggest that you take a herbal supplement that can help with these issues: it's called ashwagandha (Latin name *Withania somnifera Dunal*, and is also referred to as Indian ginseng or winter cherry). The name ashwagandha literally means 'smell of horse' – which could be because the roots of this herb do, in fact, smell like a horse; or it could be because ingesting ashwagandha makes you as strong as a horse. Take your pick!

Anxiety, depression and cortisol levels

Ashwagandha is pretty amazing stuff: it's been shown to be an effective remedy for anxiety and depression and is helpful for a host of other issues too. It basically works by modulating the amount of cortisol inside the body.

Cortisol has got itself a bad rap as the 'stress hormone', but it does a lot of other things inside us as well; the truth is that you couldn't live without it. Cortisol is a life-sustaining adrenal hormone that keeps your system in homeostasis, or balance. Cortisol has a big job to do. It has to regulate all the systems in your body relating to stress, including, but not limited to:

- Blood sugar (glucose) levels

- Fat, protein and carbohydrate metabolism to maintain blood sugar (gluconeogenesis)

- Immune responses

- Anti-inflammatory actions

- Blood pressure

- Heart and blood vessel tone and contraction

- Central nervous system activation

Cortisol levels normally go up and down, depending on the time of day. Your cortisol levels will peak about 20–30 minutes after you wake up, and reach their lowest point at around 4 a.m. This is called a circadian rhythm, and you can see the body's logic here – cortisol gets you ready to wake up in the morning by raising your blood sugar level and blood pressure, and it lowers these things at night when you're supposed to be resting.

(*Side note:* if you drink coffee, it shouldn't be consumed first thing, when you wake up, because that's when your cortisol levels are highest. Drinking coffee at peak cortisol times will lead to tolerance, and ultimately to addiction. To maximize the benefits of this caffeinated beverage, drink it between 9:30 and 11:30 a.m., when cortisol levels are dropping before the next surge. Cortisol levels normally peak in the bloodstream between 8 and 9 a.m., between noon and 1 p.m., and between 5:30 and 6:30 p.m.[1])

Of course, modern life plays havoc with our both circadian rhythm and our cortisol levels. The use of electronic lighting, computer screens, mobile phones, sugar, alcohol, and so on tends to impact our circadian rhythm – and we see this effect most strongly when we're depressed or anxious, as we're often unable to sleep properly.

Depressed people typically have problems with circadian (day-night) cortisol regulation. The normal circadian rhythm of cortisol is missing in depressed subjects – their cortisol is always raised. And this is difficult to suppress, even with normal medication.

The worst of all chronic cortisol problems stem from adverse childhood experiences: physical or sexual abuse, parents' divorce, fighting and bullying can all result in cortisol dysregulation into adulthood, including an increased risk for addiction and depression.[2]

How ashwagandha can help

In addition, the constantly high levels of stress in our culture mean that our stress response is always *on* – preventing our body from returning to 'normal' as it needs to. This can lead to health problems that stem from either too much circulating cortisol or too little cortisol if the adrenal glands become chronically tired out (adrenal fatigue).

And that's where ashwagandha comes in. In India, ashwagandha has been used in Ayurvedic medicine for thousands of years, and there's also a large amount of Western scientific literature on the herb that establishes it as one of the best, most commonly used, and extensively studied *adaptogens* available to us.

An adaptogen is something that improves our ability to cope with stress by acting on the hypothalamic-pituitary-adrenal (HPA) axis: the combination of organs in your body that deals with stress. Here's how the HPA axis works:

When you encounter a perceived threat – say, a big dog barks at you during your morning walk – your hypothalamus, a tiny region at the base of your brain, sets off an alarm system in your body. Then, like a complex game of Chinese whispers, your hypothalamus tells your pituitary, and your pituitary tells your adrenal glands, to release a surge of hormones that include adrenaline and cortisol.

Adrenaline increases your heart rate, elevates your blood pressure and boosts energy supplies. Cortisol, the primary stress hormone, increases sugars (glucose) in the bloodstream, enhances your brain's use of glucose and increases the availability of substances that repair tissues.

In a fight-or-flight situation, cortisol also shuts down any function that your brain considers 'non-essential'. (Fun fact: our brain considers our speech and language function non-essential, which is why people speaking in front of a large audience will often go blank and lose the ability to say anything at all!)

Cortisol also alters your immune system response and suppresses your digestive system, your reproductive system and your growth processes, because these things aren't considered essential when you're trying to survive an attack.

Run this entire programme occasionally, and everything will be fine – the body will return to its normal resting state once the threat has passed. But if you're in a state of chronic stress, your HPA axis basically freezes in the 'on' position. Like a car alarm that's constantly sounding, it will continuously flood your system with a stream of cortisol.

And too much cortisol, over a long period of time, will do a lot of damage inside your system. The Mayo Clinic in the USA lists that damage as follows: anxiety, depression, digestive problems, headache, heart disease, sleep problems, weight gain, and memory and concentration impairment.[3]

Studies have shown that ashwagandha actually reduces cortisol levels in the body, and can reduce severe depressive symptoms by 68 per cent. In one human study, 64 subjects suffering from chronic stress took 300mg capsules of ashwagandha or a placebo (a substance without any medicinal value) twice daily for two months.

At the end of the study period, they were asked to recomplete three questionnaires they'd answered at the beginning. The difference in the before/after scores in those questionnaires was remarkable. In the ashwagandha group[4]:

- The stress score went down by an average of 44 per cent

- The physical symptoms score decreased by 76.1 per cent

- The anxiety and insomnia score dropped by 69.7 per cent

- The social dysfunction score decreased by 68.1 per cent

- The severe depressive symptoms score dropped by 79.3 per cent

What do these figures mean? The people taking ashwagandha felt calmer and more in control. They had fewer physical symptoms of anxiety and depression, and they slept better; their productivity also increased.

The researchers concluded that 'these effects collectively suggest that ashwagandha mitigates not only the focal aspects of stress but also some of the precursors, consequences and associated symptoms of stress.

'One can think of this as ashwagandha helping both directly and indirectly. This suggests, therefore, that high-concentration, full-spectrum ashwagandha root extract possesses the ability to improve the overall wellbeing of a person.'[5]

Another study found that ashwagandha had a mood-stabilizing effect on depression and anxiety that was comparable to the antidepressants Lorazepam and Imipramine.[6]

And there's more good news: ashwagandha can help improve our sleep. Anxiety and depression block some of the body's natural coping mechanisms, and while a good night's sleep is a great stress reliever, people with these mood disorders often suffer from disrupted sleep or insomnia. And as the sleep issues can further worsen the symptoms, sufferers are caught in a vicious cycle.

Research suggests that ashwagandha can be used to ease insomnia. But it isn't a sedative: it helps us address a stress-related condition, rather than masking it with sedatives. The herb has a pronounced and positive effect on the nervous system, rejuvenating it and producing energy. This in turn eases stress and helps the body to settle back into its normal state and sleep.[7]

In another study, patients with mild to severe anxiety were given a naturopathic treatment that included ashwagandha, a multivitamin, dietary counselling and cognitive behavioural therapy (CBT). This combination seemed to have a greater effect than standard psychotherapy.[8]

Is ashwagandha safe?

According to science guidelines, an adaptogen should ideally do the following:

1. Decrease stress-induced damage.

2. Be safe and produce a beneficial effect, even if the number of administrations is more than required.

3. Be devoid of any negative effects such as withdrawal syndromes.

4. Not influence normal body functions more than necessary.

Ashwagandha does all of these things, and so is widely accepted as being beneficial and safe to use.[9] A study showed that ashwagandha is well tolerated, with few adverse side-effects. And even when the subjects were taken off the supplement abruptly at the end of the test period, none of them reported withdrawal symptoms.[10]

We have focused here on ashwagandha's effect on anxiety and depression, but it's known to have many other benefits too. There have been more than 200 studies on ashwagandha's ability to do the following:

- Improve thyroid function

- Increase stamina and endurance

- Prevent and treat cancer

- Reduce brain cell degeneration

- Stabilize blood sugar

- Lower cholesterol

- Boost immunity[11]

How to take your ashwagandha

I recommend a daily dose of 3–6 grams of dried, powdered ashwagandha root. It's beneficial to mix the powder into goat's milk (or oat/almond milk), as milk provides a nourishing base. You could put your dose in a kefir smoothie or mix it into your overnight kefir oats in the morning (see breakfast section in Chapter 11).

Ashwagandha is also available as a root extract, but I prefer the root powder – it's more difficult to overconsume and is closer to the natural form of the plant. As with any natural supplement, though, it's important to be careful and sensible when taking ashwagandha:

1. Don't go overboard with it. Although it's generally considered safe, excessive consumption could lead to stomach upset, vomiting and diarrhoea.

2. Don't consume it alongside depressants like alcohol and sedatives.

3. Don't take it in large doses if you're pregnant. Doing so may make it act like an abortifacient drug and induce miscarriage.

THE KEFIR SOLUTION SUCCESS STORY

I had IBS for more than 40 years, along with long-standing anxiety. At the time, I wasn't aware that it was IBS: back then, most of us hadn't heard of the condition. It was just something that happened to me a lot, and I simply got on with it. I don't think I realized how debilitating it was.

I recently asked my daughter what she remembered about my IBS from when she was a child. 'You were always tired,' she said. That was hard to hear, because it's important to me that I was a good mother to her.

But I was always tired, and I always struggled with eating. My symptoms led to a lot of social anxiety, too: in fact, it got to the point where I couldn't go out of the house, even into the garden. I was anxious about everything.

Things got really bad when my daughter was about 10 years old. I had no ability to handle crises. I couldn't go outside for three months and was off work for nine months. Driving on the motorway was difficult, and I struggled when travelling – it's a bit like when you're potty training a child, and you always need to know the location of the nearest toilet.

I saw a doctor, who prescribed peppermint. I also tried acupuncture and aloe vera, and took Naproxin for the pain. These all worked for a time, but then they stopped. While I was looking for something else that might help, I saw Chuckling Goat featured on the TV show Countrywise, and I thought I'd have a go with the kefir.

The first thing that went was the bloating. Then I started feeling that I had a bit more energy and could go out and walk, which is important to me. You don't realize how much IBS's constant low level of discomfort affects you – until it goes away.

I stopped feeling queasy from the bloating all the time: that really helped! I felt more confident, and was able to use public transport. It sounds a bit crazy, but it's really useful to be able to take the train without having to take Diazepam to cope with the anxiety! I could start going out to concerts, too.

Now I'm more relaxed. Taking the kefir allows me to have a life, without just doing the bare minimum. We all need a life with more depth and variety in it. I would recommend Chuckling Goat kefir to anyone.

GILL DOVE, 57, PROOFREADER, CUMBRIA, UK

Chapter 8

The Kefir Solution Step #3: Lean in to Your Feelings

When you're working with IBS, depression and anxiety, strong, often negative emotions are obviously a huge part of the mix. You now know a little about the neuroscience of your emotions: what's happening inside your brain and gut to create the feelings that you're feeling.

Any emotion that you're experiencing right now is essentially a wash of neurochemicals flooding through your body and affecting all your organs, moment to moment. It has a lot to do with the way that your body is processing the neurotransmitter serotonin (see Chapter 3) and how your gut bugs are functioning.

But until the Kefir Solution takes effect and you get better, *you'll still be feeling what you're feeling*. It's funny, isn't it, that knowing *why* you're feeling something doesn't keep you from experiencing it; not one bit. You still have those strong emotions.

Introducing emotion recognition

Here in the West, we have a strange relationship with our emotions. We particularly try to avoid negative emotions: in fact, we'll do just about *anything* not to feel those – drink, take drugs, shop, watch TV, gamble. Addiction is largely fuelled by this desire to avoid our negative emotions.

So here's a radical, revolutionary and somewhat scary concept – what if you were to actually *lean in* to your emotions, and pull them towards you, like weights in a gym? I call this practice 'emotion recognition', and it involves moving towards your emotions instead of trying to push them away. It's a discipline, and you work it like a muscle.

What emotion recognition means, ultimately, is that your emotions are okay. It's okay to have them, and it's okay to feel them. In fact, you *need* to feel them, for the sake of your emotional wellbeing.

To work with your depression and anxiety effectively, you actually need to *feel* the sadness, rather than push it away. Sounds crazy, but the quickest way is through! *Feeling your feelings* **will help you get through them quicker, and out the other side.**

The latest science demonstrates that emotion recognition can help you to become more resilient. When difficult things happen, you'll still experience sadness, but your system will recover faster – just as an athlete's cardiovascular system recovers more quickly than that of someone who sits on the couch all day.

Accepting your emotions

According to new research reported in the *Journal of Personality and Social Psychology*, embracing our darker emotions, rather than trying to escape them, is more likely to benefit our psychological health in the long term.

In a study of more than 1,300 adults, researchers found that subjects who reported trying to avoid negative emotions in response to bad experiences were more likely to have symptoms of mood disorders, such as anxiety and depression, six months later, compared with those who embraced their negative emotions.[1]

Seems strange, right? But it turns out it's all about *acceptance*. This is true whether the issue is embracing our good or bad attributes or accepting the way we look – or the way we feel.

In the study, the research team set out to determine how acceptance of negative emotions – such as sadness, disappointment and anger – might influence psychological health. The participants completed a survey in which they were asked to rate how strongly they agreed with certain statements, such as, 'I tell myself I shouldn't be feeling the way that I'm feeling.'

In three different experiments, researchers found that participants who had lower agreement with such statements as these – indicating a greater acceptance of negative feelings – showed higher levels of psychological wellbeing, compared with subjects who attempted to resist negative feelings. They also found that participants who tried to avoid feeling negativity about certain tasks were more likely to experience distress, compared with subjects who embraced any negative feelings.

'We found that people who habitually accept their negative emotions experience fewer negative emotions, which adds up to better psychological health,' says senior study author Iris Mauss, an associate professor of psychology at the University of California, Berkeley.

'Overall, the team believes that when bad things happen, it may be better to let negative emotions run their course rather than trying to avoid them. It turns out that how we approach our own negative emotional reactions is really important for our overall wellbeing. People who accept these emotions without judging or trying to change them are able to cope with their stress more successfully.'[2]

I know that leaning in to your feelings in this way may seem strange. And unfamiliar. And frightening. And it's probably the last thing you want to do when you're feeling anxious and depressed. But it is, in fact, *what works*.

Our time-honoured, knee-jerk reaction of trying to avoid our feelings just doesn't work to make us feel better. And if you keep doing what you've always done, you're just going to get the results you've always had.

✿ EMOTION RECOGNITION IN ACTION ✿

So, are you willing to give emotion recognition a try? Here's how you can start practising it right this minute.

⟡ Imagine that you're turning directly towards whatever emotion you're experiencing right now, until it's immediately in front of you. Take a moment to perceive it. Does it have a colour, a weight, a shape, a texture? Is it sharp or dull?

⟡ Now inhale that emotion straight into your heart, breathing in deeply through your nose. That's right: it seems counterintuitive and crazy, but it won't harm you. Just suck that feeling straight into you.

✤ At the top of your in-held breath, pause for a moment and think of all the other people in the world who are feeling exactly the same thing as you are right now. There are millions of them out there! Then exhale slowly through your mouth, silently saying the word 'peace', with the intention of creating peace for yourself and for everyone else.

✤ Complete the third step three times. The second time, breathe out 'serenity'. And the third time, exhale 'strength' – for yourself and everyone else.

✤ Continue with this practice until your perception of the emotion begins to shift. If you wish, you can continue the experience, working with this new perception. How has it shifted? What's the colour, weight, shape and texture of the emotion now?

✤ Inhale this new emotion into your heart. Pause to connect with all the millions of people out there who are feeling exactly the same thing as you are right this minute. Then exhale slowly through your mouth, silently saying peace, then serenity and then strength – for yourself and for everyone else.

🌀 🌀 🌀

This practice allows you to assimilate your emotions so that you can absorb them – just as you chew up food in order to digest it. Same process.

Emotion recognition with others

You can practise emotion recognition with those around you as well. Instead of trying to 'cheer up' a person or fix their problem, try just agreeing with them: 'Wow, that *is* really sad. I would feel sad too.' Then just sit with them while they experience their emotion.

That's it! Simple, but incredibly difficult at the same time – because it's exactly the opposite of what we're used to. And revolutionary: as you'll find out if you start putting emotion recognition to work in your life.

Here's another example of the practice in action. Imagine that a child has lost a treasured teddy bear: maybe it's been left on the train, and is now gone for good. Tears and panic! Can you feel an impulse rising in you to distract, to diminish, to try to buy the child off with something? What are the things we normally say, in a situation like that?

'Come on now, don't cry.' (Just deny your feelings.)

'If you're good, I'll buy you another teddy.' (Hello, online shopping habit.)

'Cheer up: have a cookie!' (Learn to squash your feelings by consuming sugar.)

'What a big fuss about nothing. That teddy was old anyway.' (Your feelings aren't valid. It's wrong to be sad.)

Imagine that, instead of saying these things, you just sit with the child and agree with their feelings: acknowledging the rightness of them. What if you even help them put words to their feelings? They'll still feel sad, but at least they won't feel *alone*. Feeling isolated is one of the worst things about experiencing pain.

What if you say, 'I can see that you feel sad. I would feel sad too. It's really hard, when you lose something you love.' And then imagine that you just sit there, offering your support while the child works their way through and processes their feelings.

I've done this with my own children, and I can tell you that it produces startling results. They are now more emotionally *resilient*. Like an athlete in training whose heart rate rapidly returns to normal after exercise, children trained in emotion recognition recover more quickly. Sure, they still feel sad when bad things happen – but they *bounce*.

Emotion recognition in business

You can take this knowledge to work with you, as well. I use emotion recognition in every aspect of my business, Chuckling Goat. We don't ask our employees to leave their feelings at the door: we instruct them to bring them in. We're all about authenticity, and we believe that gold star leadership involves being courageous enough to let your team *see your emotions*.

Why does this work? Well, imagine a typical CEO of a Fortune 500 business. Which emotions would you imagine he or she would express, or permit, in the workplace? When I asked my team this question, they suggested aggression, anger, power, dominance, intimidation and irritation.

That's hardly the full, rich spectrum of human emotion, is it? In fact, most of them aren't emotions at all: they're just strategies for controlling people. We've long associated emotions with being weak, unprofessional, hysterical and feminine. As a young reporter, I was upset after receiving some hate mail, and I went to ask my female boss for advice. Her response? 'Get a thicker skin.'

The adjective *businesslike* is commonly used as the antithesis of emotional. *It's just business* is a phrase that's often used to justify some horrific betrayal.

And yet... and yet...

At Chuckling Goat, emotion recognition has played a big part in our success. Why?

Because until now, the traditional business world has got it all wrong when it comes to emotion. Literally 180 degree, upside-down wrong. There's a pivotal piece of information that's been missing from the equation, and it's why we should be embracing emotion in business rather than leaving it at the door: *emotion is the major driver of human decision-making.*

This is the dirty secret of the human brain: you make your decisions not on the logical side of your brain, but on the emotional side. The logical side of your brain can build up arguments all day long, but the actual moment of decision comes from the emotional side: the side that deals with humour, colour and narrative.

Scientists know this because of the ground-breaking work of Antonio Damasio. This Portuguese-American neurologist worked with a successful lawyer called 'Elliot', who underwent surgery on the right side of his brain to remove a tumour.

After the surgery, Elliot was able to function normally in many ways, but he could no longer make even the simplest decisions. The arguments would stack up endlessly, but the magical moment of choosing would never occur. It couldn't: because the emotional side of his brain had been damaged.[3]

You can use logic and reason and make pro-con lists all day long, but at the end of the day, it's the emotional side of your brain that drives you to actual action – including the decision to purchase a product. That's just how decisions are made.

Customers buy from companies that they know, like and trust, because they decide to purchase something *based on emotion*. Fail to connect with your customers, and your business will fail. Connect successfully using narrative and emotion, and your business will explode – as ours has done.

And when a manager is brave enough to bring his or her emotions into the workplace – in a vulnerable, authentic way – it creates a sense of loyalty among the team that makes them *unbreakable*. Alignment is the Holy Grail of management, and employees don't align to a robotic, aggressive, controlling leader. They align with a real human being whom they trust.

Emotion recognition in a nutshell

So here's a summary of the practice:

Myth It's best to avoid or deny your negative emotions, and keep a 'stiff upper lip'.

Fact People who *accept* their negative emotions actually experience *fewer* negative emotions, and recover from them faster.

Myth Emotion has no place in business.

Fact Decisions are made on the emotional side of the brain. Customers buy from brands they know, like and trust. Team members align to leaders who authentically show their emotions, and demonstrate that they're trustworthy.

It's all about emotion. So, validate those emotions at home and at work – for yourself, for your family, for your team and for your customers!

Crying is good for you!

Another way to work with your anxiety and depression is to release your feelings by crying. Crying is good for you, and it makes you feel better faster, so go for it! Cry at every possible opportunity. Crying is your body's way of purging the neurochemicals of depression and emotion from your system, and if you don't do it, those chemicals will remain and create disease and dysfunction.

Did you know that you have different kinds of tears? One kind is a lubricant and functions simply to keep your eyes moist. But emotional, or weeping, tears are formed when you experience great joy or sorrow. Any powerful emotional response may generate these tears, including anger.

Emotional tears have a different chemical composition than lubricating tears: they contain stress hormones and other toxins that accumulate during stress. Releasing these chemicals from your system in the form of tears is your body's way of purging them.

William Frey, a biochemist and director of the Psychiatry Research Laboratories at St Paul-Ramsey Medical Center in the USA commented on his research into the biological role emotional tears play in health:

'People say they feel better after crying, and our data show this is so. Crying is an exocrine process. That is, a process in which a substance comes out of the body. Other exocrine processes, like exhaling, urinating, defecating and sweating, release toxic substances from the body. There's every reason to think that crying does the same, releasing chemicals that the body produces in response to stress.'[4]

So the emotional shedding of tears has healing power as it helps to release powerful emotional triggers, including stress, anger, sadness, grief and joy. Crying may also stimulate your body to produce endorphins: 'feel-good' hormones that help balance your emotional state. Even when the emotional or situational problem persists, crying may help you feel better and improve your decisions about that situation.[5]

Pleasure versus happiness: making choices

I'd like to make an important point here: one that isn't made very often in our society. It's about the distinction between *pleasure* and *happiness*.

Aren't they the same thing? No, they're absolutely not. As endocrinologist Robert H. Lustig explains in his book *The Hacking of the American Mind: The Science Behind the Corporate Takeover of Our Bodies and Brains,* biochemically speaking, pleasure and happiness are two completely different things. And understanding why could change your life forever.

What is pleasure?

The sensation of pleasure is created by a neurotransmitter called dopamine. Remember neurotransmitters – the chemicals that neurons release in order to communicate with one another? Well, dopamine is one of those, along with serotonin.

Dopamine creates a 'reward-generating' pathway in your brain that delivers the same sensation of pleasure *regardless* of the source of that pleasure. Pick your stimulus: it can be an activity, like pornography, shopping, gambling or surfing the Internet. It can be a food, or alcohol or drugs. Whatever the source, the dopamine pleasure kick produced is the same.[6]

What's the problem with this? Dopamine is a 'poisoned chalice' substance, which means the more you get, the more you want. It's a so-called *excitatory neurotransmitter*, and too much of it is neurotoxic – meaning that, over time, it causes cell death.

When one neuron releases dopamine and another neuron accepts the signal, it can damage the receiving neuron. To protect itself from damage, the neuron receiving the signal downregulates (reduces or suppresses) its receptors. (If you were a neuron, you would do the same!)

Result? Fewer receptors on the receiving neuron mean that the dopamine has less effect. Every time you get a 'hit' of dopamine, the number of receptors decreases. As a result, you need increasingly larger 'hits' to get the same effect. Eventually, you end up with 'tolerance': a state in which even a large dose produces no effect. Once the neurons actually start to die off, you're a full-blown addict.[7]

One quick and easy way to stimulate dopamine is to eat sugar. That's why you may reach for a chocolate bar when you feel down, imagining that it will give you a boost. Neurochemically, however, this is impossible. Sugar will give you a temporary dopamine pleasure rush, but it will never, ever – for reasons we'll discuss shortly – make you *happy*.

Add the stress hormone cortisol to the mix, which downregulates serotonin, and what do you get then? Addiction and depression.[8] Look around any city in the world and you'll see this illustrated in more ways than you can count. It takes up to three weeks for the dopamine receptors to repopulate and if an individual is really addicted, the cravings can go on for more than a year.[9]

What is happiness?

Now let's talk about serotonin. While dopamine causes pleasure, serotonin causes the sensation of happiness, or contentment. Serotonin is *not* an excitatory neurotransmitter. When serotonin acts on its receptor, no damage occurs. So happiness, or contentment, does *not* lead to addictive behaviour.

But here's the real kicker: dopamine downregulates serotonin. So the more *pleasure* you have, the less *happiness* you're going to feel, and the more 'hits' you're going to need, just to keep the pleasure level up. What does this mean for you? Basically, it means that it's impossible to achieve lasting happiness (serotonin) by engaging in pleasure-seeking behaviour (dopamine).[10]

And we can add to this the fact that, as we've already discussed, to make serotonin you need an amino acid called tryptophan, which is found only in food. If you remember, tryptophan is a precursor (a substance from which another substance is formed) for serotonin.

Tryptophan is like a teenager without a car: it has to ride-share its amino acid transporter with two other common amino acids called phenylalanine and tyrosine. What do these two amino acids do? They are precursors to dopamine.

You can't have both dopamine and serotonin – because they compete for resources and cancel each other out. *You have to choose.* This is why addicts aren't happy people. Explains an awful lot, don't you think?

Tryptophan and the brain

So, let's imagine for a moment that you're going to opt for serotonin instead of dopamine. (And I sincerely hope that you are!) Let's look at how we can get more serotonin into your life. As you know, to make serotonin, you need to eat high-tryptophan foods. But there are three challenges with that:[11]

- Tryptophan is one of the rarest amino acids in our diet: eggs contain the most; poultry has some; there's very little in vegetables; and carbohydrates have none.

- Even if you do manage to get it into your system, 99.9 per cent of the tryptophan you ingest either gets turned into serotonin in the gut for your gut's purposes, or it goes into your platelets (tiny blood cells) to helps them clot. So there's very little tryptophan left over to make its way to the brain.

- Eating too much processed food makes everything worse because processing tends to deplete food of tryptophan, as well as clogging up your amino acid transporters with dopamine precursors.

So, getting that all-important tryptophan into your system isn't easy – which is why we don't all feel happy every moment of every day. But it *can* be done! We're going to take a look at the foods that contain tryptophan in the next chapter. But there are other methods of boosting your serotonin levels, and some of them may surprise you!

In his book *The Hacking of the American Mind*, Robert H. Lustig outlines some non-dietary ways to get serotonin into your life. He argues that it's your experiences that make you happy. People can make you happy, too, and you can make yourself happier.

✿ FOUR WAYS TO MAKE YOURSELF HAPPY ✿

According to Robert H. Lustig, there are four key ways to make yourself happy by boosting your serotonin levels, and they're all free:[12]

1: CONNECT

Make genuine human connections. Communicating on social media doesn't count, because interpersonal connection means eye-to-eye contact. Seeing the expressions of the person to whom you're speaking activates a set of neurons in your brain called mirror neurons, which are the drivers of empathy and specifically linked to serotonin.

This doesn't happen online; in fact, it's just the opposite: use of social media generates dopamine, which leads to addiction, and reduces happiness. So online connection is another 'poisoned chalice' solution that ends up driving unhappiness.

2: CONTRIBUTE

Be part of something greater than yourself: make a contribution to society. For example, scientific research shows that volunteering improves depression, life satisfaction and wellbeing, as well as resulting in a 22 per cent reduction in the risk of death.

3: COPE

Poor sleep, lack of exercise and multitasking are all causes of unhappiness. Sleep is very important for healthy serotonin production. Avoiding exposure to the blue light emitted by electronic screens is essential, as this inhibits melatonin production, making it harder to sleep.

4: COOK

Eat real food that you've prepared yourself. If you cook, you're more likely to increase your tryptophan intake, reduce the amount of refined sugar you eat, and increase your anti-inflammatory omega-3 fats and fibre (more on these coming up). Overall, this benefits your gut bugs, which in turn will increase serotonin levels in your system.

❀ ❀ ❀

Love your tummy

Here's a weird question for you: do you love your tummy? If you don't, you're not alone. Women in particular carry a huge amount of shame about their midsection. Maybe you think your tummy is too fat, has too many stretchmarks and is too squidgy. Add in the IBS – with all the bloating and the gurgling and the pain – and like the relationship status option on Facebook, *it's complicated.*

But here's the thing: all that tension, holding-in, discomfort, resentment and irritation that you may be directing towards your midsection is really just making everything worse.

All of those emotions create cortisol inside the system, and cortisol is a happiness killer. Cortisol is the anti-contentment hormone.

Contentment means all is well and it's okay to relax. Your body figures – and rightly so – that if the adrenal glands are releasing cortisol, something must be wrong.

Cortisol has a huge biochemical impact on how you're feeling, as well. It wipes out your gut bugs: like a tidal wave sweeping through the Amazon rainforest. As we've already discussed, over time, raised cortisol levels can contribute to anxiety, depression and digestive problems – the constellation of issues we're trying to get on top of. So 'tummy hatred' is just locking you further into the vicious spiral of bad feeling and feeling bad.

The first place we feel nerves, fear or anxiety is in our stomach. We spend a lot of time holding in our tummies, or trying to flatten them. And when you experience tummy-hatred, it raises your cortisol levels and damages your digestion. This will contribute to abdominal discomfort as your digestive function slows down. The microbial diversity of your gut bugs will be reduced, further decreasing your bugs' ability to digest and absorb your food.

So, how do we get out of this nasty cycle? The solution is the same as for nearly any other challenge you can think of – love. You're going to have to start loving your own tum. *Impossible: that relationship is broken*, you might say. You might think that your tummy has let you down too many times, and that there's just too much bad history between you.

How about starting with gratitude? Your tummy does a lot for you, you know. If your body stopped working on its own tomorrow, what would you miss the most about today? Try the following exercise right now:

✺ SHOW GRATITUDE TOWARDS YOUR TUMMY ✺

✧ Lean back, close your eyes and place your hands over your belly. Feel the warmth of your hands there.

✧ Breathe into your hands, so that your hands – and belly – expand on the in-breath and fall back into place on the out-breath.

✧ Do this three or four times. And then say in your head (or out loud, if you're brave enough!): *I'm sorry. I love you. Forgive me. Thank you.*

✧ Repeat this over and over. If you feel a bit teary, that's fine – let it come. It's not surprising to feel emotional when you reconnect with a forgotten, hidden and hated part of yourself. After all, how do you think your tummy feels? It's been doing its best for you all these years and what has it got in return, besides abuse and resentment? Time to mend those tummy fences.

✺ ✺ ✺

Another great way to repair the relationship with your tummy is to give yourself an abdominal massage. Sound strange? It shouldn't, as we routinely get a massage for our back, shoulders and neck. But that unloved bit of ourselves, our tummy, misses out again.

✺ GIVE YOURSELF AN ABDOMINAL MASSAGE ✺

I recommend that you perform this simple massage twice daily, once when you wake up, and then again just before you go to sleep. Close your eyes as you massage, and repeat your tummy-love mantra: *I'm sorry. I love you. Forgive me. Thank you.*

✤ Lie flat on your back on a firm bed or on a mat placed on the floor.

✤ Expose your belly by lifting up your top: this is so you can get skin-to-skin contact with your tummy.

✤ Rub your hands against one another firmly for about 15 seconds, until they feel very warm.

✤ Place three fingers into your navel and begin a very gentle, firm (but not painful) rubbing motion. Slowly circle outwards from the navel, moving clockwise: this echoes the direction of the large intestine.

✤ Focus your mind on the warmth building up in your abdominal area as you continue the motion for two minutes – during which time you'll have made 40 or 50 circles on your tummy.

᪥ ᪥ ᪥

That's it! You've just performed your first abdominal massage. Your tummy will respond to the loving attention you pay it!

Chapter 9

The Kefir Solution Step #4: Alter Your Eating Habits

We've now explored how taking kefir and ashwagandha and dealing with your feelings can help. Now it's time to examine the biggie – your eating habits.

This can be a difficult and emotional topic. Chances are that you've tried loads of diets: the average 45-year-old woman in the UK has been on 61 diets.[1] It can be incredibly dispiriting and disheartening to try diet after diet, and have nothing ever work.

But the eating principles we're going to discuss now are not a 'diet'. This step in the programme is not something that you're going to pick up for a few weeks, lose a few pounds and then drop; instead, it's a way of eating differently for life.

Does what we eat affect the gut–brain axis?

So before we begin, is it worth investing your time and energy into changing your eating patterns? Can the dietary aspects of the

Kefir Solution, which include eating certain foods while avoiding others, *really* help heal your IBS, anxiety and depression? Science ᴄᴀʏᴇ ᴊᴇᴇ and let's quickly recap on why.

In 2013, researchers at the University of California, Los Angeles (UCLA) discovered the first hard evidence that bacteria ingested in food can affect the human brain. During a four-week study, they found that the participants who consumed a dairy product containing probiotics twice daily showed altered brain function; this was seen both while they were in a resting state *and* as they responded to a task that looked at their emotional reaction to a visual stimulus.

As you now know, scientists have long since discovered that the brain sends signals to the gut, which is why stress and other emotions can contribute to gastrointestinal symptoms. But in the UCLA study, researchers were amazed to discover something we've been discussing in this book: the signals travel the opposite way as well, and *changing the microbiota in the gut can affect the brain*.

'Time and time again, we hear from patients that they never felt depressed or anxious until they started experiencing problems with their gut,' says Dr Kirsten Tillisch, an associate professor of medicine at UCLA's David Geffen School of Medicine and a lead author of the study. 'Our study shows that the gut–brain connection is a two-way street.'[2]

The researchers were surprised to find that the brain effects could be seen in many areas, including those involved in sensory processing, and not merely those associated with emotion.

Dr Emeran Mayer, the study's senior author, says: 'There are studies showing that what we eat can alter the composition and products of the gut flora – in particular, that people with high-vegetable, fibre-based diets have a different composition of their microbiota, or gut environment, than people who eat the more typical Western diet that is high in (saturated) fat and carbohydrates. Now we know that this has an effect not only on the metabolism but also on brain function.[3]

So the UCLA study, and many others, confirms that in order to heal your IBS, depression and anxiety, you need to heal your microbiome.

Imagine now that I've waved a wand over you, made you tiny and inserted you inside your own gut. You're wandering through a landscape containing all kinds of crazy flora and fauna. But this landscape is blasted and stunted. As in the Yellowstone National Park story, some of the key players have been removed, and there has been a trophic cascade of disastrous events. The ecosystem is falling apart.

We need to do some repair work in here, some 'restorative ecology'. Think of yourself as a relief worker to the environment. You're going to plant trees, refurbish habitats, remove sources of poison and pollution, and get those streams running clean and restocked with fish. We're going to put the wolves back into Yellowstone.

In this scenario, you can think of kefir as the wolves. Taking kefir is the big stroke that's going to create change inside your system. But kefir on its own is not enough. You also have to support the action of the kefir inside your system. So, how are we going to do this? Mainly with food.

A new way to think about food

In order to accomplish your objective, I need you to start thinking differently about food, both *what* you eat and *why* you eat it. As I said earlier, this step in the Kefir Solution is not a 'diet': it's educational principles about how the environment inside you functions.

Once you know these things, *you know them forever*. If you go into a blasted landscape and painstakingly work to restore the ecosystem, do you then turn around and order more bleach to pour into the rivers? Of course not: you respect both the environment and all the hard work that you've done to restore it.

It's just the same inside your microbiome. Over the next nine weeks or so, during the initial process of getting started with the Kefir Solution, you're going to put in some hard work to reclaim your inner ecosystem.

And once that work is done, you'll need to continue to respect and care for that environment. Can you have treats, once your health has been restored? Sure. But be aware that they're *treats*, and should only be enjoyed now and then.

And until you're feeling in good shape again, you need to be pretty strict. Reclaiming a blasted landscape is not easy, and the kefir can't do all the work on its own.

So let's think about this: why do you eat? To stay alive? Because you're hungry? Because you're bored? Because you're trying to push away an emotion that you don't want to deal with? Because you have a craving? Because you fancy something?

Eating to feed your 'good' gut bugs

I'm going to suggest a new motivation for your eating: to feed the good bugs in your microbiome.

Remember that you're a symbiont: a constellation of human and non-human cells. Inside you are cells that make up human tissues and organs, and then a bunch of non-human cells, or microbes – bacteria, viruses, fungi and archaea. The human cells and non-human cells are coexisting inside the same symbiont – that's you.

Coexisting with your gut bugs means that you strike a deal with them: they produce energy and vitamins, and help screen out pathogens that threaten your human cells. In return, your human cells help maintain the microbial habit, providing them with a stable environment in which they can thrive and grow.

Classic win-win! Once you understand how your microbiome works, you no longer have only yourself to please. It's not just about you and what your tongue wants to taste. You have a responsibility to all of those trillions of tiny critters in there. They have needs. And just because you're bigger than they are, and you happen to control the mouth, it doesn't mean that you get to ignore those needs. Nor are your bugs going to *allow you* to ignore them.

In fact, the IBS, depression and anxiety you're experiencing are all ways in which your gut bugs are responding to what you've been feeding them, and the things to which you've been exposing them. Remember: *this is a two-way street.*

'Our gut microbes are not just passive recipients of the food that we eat – they evolve and change in response to what we feed our bodies,' says Athena Aktipis, a researcher at Arizona State University's Biodesign Institute in the USA.

'There are certain foods that lead to resource sharing between us and our microbes, while other foods can lead to conflict and resource competition between our bodies and our microbes. This cooperation and conflict framework can help us understand certain aspects of why we get sick and how we can stay healthy.'[4]

Your gut bugs are living organisms, and like all living organisms, they are constantly evolving. But *how* will they evolve? That's up to you, because when it comes to your gut bugs, *you* are the forces of evolution!

Why your food choices matter

The two processes that determine evolution are competition and cooperation. And the road down which your gut bugs travel is determined by the food *you* choose to eat. Your dietary decisions determine your bugs' destiny, and dictate whether they will live or die, cooperate or compete.

But the plot gets even thicker, because you control your bugs' destiny, and *they control yours*. The choice of conflict or cooperation between your cells means the difference between your being healthy or ill. One example of cells that compete is cancer cells, which mutate genetically, form independent clusters and rob resources from the host for their own benefit.

Can you see why your decisions around what foods to eat need to be driven by something larger than whether or not you happen to fancy something in that particular moment? There are many lives at stake here, and one of them is yours!

So what should happen? You need to *align* the needs of your gut microbes with your own needs. Alignment leads to positive health outcomes. Conflict over resources generates disease.

(*Side note*: I can't help but see comparisons with the political situation of the larger ecosystem on Planet Earth. The more research I do in this area, the more I'm convinced it's all a fractal – the pattern is the same inside us, or outside us. And the ultimate solutions are the same: align and cooperate, don't compete!)

Just think of things from a microbial point of view. How can you and your gut bugs get on the same page? Internal disputes break out when you and your microbes are at cross-purposes. And when the conditions of cooperation break down, the result is IBS, anxiety and depression. Plus a whole host of other nasty health issues.

So what *causes* this internal conflict? You won't be surprised by the answer: eating foods that are low in fibre and high in simple sugars (carbohydrates that burn quickly inside your body, producing a rapid increase in blood sugar), saturated fats and emulsifying agents. And this includes most processed foods.

If there's too much sugar and too little fibre in your diet, the population of 'bad' bugs living in your gut explodes. Your body will respond by ramping up immune activity against them, which can result in an escalating conflict between your human and your microbial cells that will have disastrous effects on your health.

Foods that are high in nutrients and low in harmful elements (such as salmon, kale, liver, sweet potatoes, sardines, blueberries, broccoli and eggs) act in the opposite way: they foster cooperation between your human cells and your microbial ones.

And the non-digestible carbohydrates in milk kefir feed the protective bugs in the gut. The specialized proteins in kefir also provide an immunological effect, including cytokines, immunoglobulins and lactoferrin that act to reduce infection risk.

This is a real departure from conventional ideas about diet. To sum up: what you eat affects the subtle interconnection between host (you) and microbiome. Essentially, you've got to feed the *right population* of gut bugs.[5] It makes me think of a Native American story in which an old Cherokee teaches his grandson about life:

'A fight is going on inside me. It's a terrible fight and it's between two wolves,' the old man says to the boy.

'One is evil – he is anger, envy, sorrow, regret, greed, arrogance, self-pity, guilt, resentment, inferiority, lies, false pride, superiority, and ego. The other is good – he is joy, peace, love, hope, serenity, humility, kindness, benevolence, empathy, generosity, truth, compassion and faith.

'The same fight is going on inside you – and inside every other person, too.'

The boy thought about his grandfather's words for a minute and then asked him: 'Which wolf will win?'

The old Cherokee replies, 'The one you feed.'

So, which wolf are *you* going to feed?

Promoting tolerance inside the gut

So we now know that we need to choose our foods with more intention, in order to feed the right population of gut bacteria. We know that sugar, and processed foods that are low in fibre and high in unhealthy fats, feed the bad bugs. But what about the 'good' bugs? Who are they, and what do they like to eat?

Inside your gut, 'human' immune cells are on patrol, protecting you from harmful microbes lurking in the food you eat. Some are hardcore, SAS-type fighter cells that are ready to cause inflammation if they find a troublemaker. These warriors are balanced out by immune cells that promote tolerance: they protect the body from pathogens without damaging its sensitive tissues.[6]

But your 'human' immune system cells and the symbiotic 'bugs' in your gut are inextricably linked, and there's no meaningful way to tease them apart. It's now been established that the bosses of your immune system – the T-cells – actually take *their* marching orders from the symbiotic bugs. So when it comes to your immune system, the bugs are really running the show![7]

As ever in your gut, the balance is delicate. Tip things too far towards inflammation, and you end up with trouble. So we want to foster more of those tolerance-promoting bugs.

Recent research on mice by the Washington University School of Medicine in the USA found that high levels of our old friend tryptophan, in the presence of a bacterial species called *Lactobacillus* (which is found in kefir), may cause expansion in this population of tolerance-promoting cells.

When the researchers doubled the amount of tryptophan in the mice's feed, the number of such cells rose by about 50 per cent. When tryptophan levels were halved, the number of cells dropped by half.

Humans have the same tolerance-promoting immune cells as mice, and most of us shelter *Lactobacillus* in our gastrointestinal tracts.[8] So, long story short – the combination of *Lactobacillus* and a tryptophan-rich diet may foster a more tolerant, less inflammatory gut environment.

THE KEFIR SOLUTION SUCCESS STORY

I developed IBS seven years ago, after my husband passed away. We were one of those very lucky couples: we were very fond of each other, and losing him was very difficult. I was in a lot of pain, and had 'explosions' each morning: I couldn't go out before 10:30 a.m.

After I started taking the kefir, I saw a remarkable difference within the first week. I followed all the instructions, including switching to goat's cheese, milk and butter, etc. I found all that very helpful.

The pain disappeared and my bowels became more regular. I was so pleased. I've also lost a lot of weight, which I'm happy about: the steroids I'd been taking had made my tummy bloat. Recently, a friend told me they'd never seen me looking better. Definitely, without a shadow of a doubt, the Kefir Solution has made me feel so much better. I think my skin's even improved.

DIANA C., 83, RETIRED DOCTOR'S RECEPTIONIST,
NORTH YORKSHIRE, UK

Chapter 10

The Kefir Solution
Eating Principles

So, you're starting to build a picture of the types of food you need to eat in order to raise those serotonin levels inside your system, and combat your IBS, anxiety and depression. These can be summarized as three eating principles:

1. Feed your good bugs, which you'll introduce to your gut by drinking kefir.

2. Starve your bad bugs.

3. Don't irritate your gut.

Let's now look at each principle in turn.

Feed your good bugs: eat tryptophan-rich foods

In order to make serotonin, your body needs tryptophan, which as you now know, is found only in food. When you think tryptophan, think *protein-rich foods*: nuts, eggs, seeds, beans, fish, chicken, turkey, lamb, beef, pork, yogurt, cheese. Chocolate also contains tryptophan (but before you get all crazy, it's found only in dark chocolate, with 70 per cent cocoa solids or higher).

Interestingly, studies have found that people's trust in others – a serotonin-mediated function – increased after they ate tryptophan-rich foods. It really does work![1]

Try to include more of the following tryptophan-rich foods in your diet:

- Free-range eggs (especially the whites)

- Spirulina

- Wild-caught fish, such as cod and salmon, rather than farmed fish

- Pasture-raised poultry

- Grass-fed beef or lamb

- Goat's milk, goat's yogurt, goat's cheese

- Sesame seeds, cashew nuts and walnuts

- 100 per cent wholegrain oats, or quinoa

- Soaked or sprouted legumes, including beans, chickpeas and peas

- New or sweet potatoes

- Bananas

The following foods contain less tryptophan than those listed previously, but are still good sources for those following a vegan or vegetarian diet:

- Soya (soy): soya beans/soybeans are an excellent source of protein; in fact, they are the only vegetable with a complete protein. However, I recommend that you choose organic fermented soya – the type that's been used in many Asian cultures for thousands of years. Think nattō, miso, tempeh, and organic, fermented, traditionally made soy sauce.

  It's best to *avoid unfermented* soya products, such as fresh soya beans, dried soya beans, soya nuts, soya sprouts, soya flour, soya milk, tofu and the soya protein found in most protein powders.

- Pumpkin

- Cauliflower

- Cucumber

- Mushrooms

- Green leafy vegetables

Choose eggs for tryptophan

I'd like to say a word in defence of eggs, which have taken a bit of a beating on the reputation front in recent years. Eggs are a magic food, so eat them!

For the purpose of our IBS-depression-anxiety discussion, the best thing about eggs is that they are a great source of tryptophan. But eggs are good for loads of other things as well. In the words of Dr Natasha Campbell McBride, the doyenne of gut science and health, author of *Gut and Psychology Syndrome* and founder of the GAPS diet:

'Eggs are one of the most nourishing and easy ways to digest foods on this planet. Raw egg yolk has been compared with human breast milk because it can be absorbed almost 100 per cent without needing digestion. Egg yolks will provide you with most essential amino acids, many vitamins (B1, B2, B12, A, D, biotin), essential fatty acids, a lot of zinc, magnesium and many other nutrients.'

Or, in the words of my 12-year-old son: 'Yum!' On the farm, we're lucky to have our own chickens. There's nothing so lovely as cracking a farm fresh egg into the pan, and seeing that gorgeous deep yellow yolk that comes from a happy chicken that's been wandering around the farm, pecking for bugs and hunting for goodies.

We eat eggs almost every day. Although we start with an early breakfast of overnight kefir oats (see recipe in Chapter 11) before the morning chores, we usually take a break around 11 a.m. for a big, protein-rich plate of scrambled eggs. We work hard on the farm, and we're hungry by then.

In fact, early afternoon is actually the best time to have your protein, as your body processes heavy fats and proteins better during the day than after 6 p.m. If I'm trying to shift a bit of weight, I have all my protein earlier in the day. I then swap my supper for a green smoothie, which I sip while everyone else is having their meal (*see the Super Supper Smoothie recipe on page 181*).

We add other goodies to our scrambled eggs: our favourite combinations are salmon, soft goat's cheese and leek, or chicken, avocado and hard goat's cheese. Just toss the ingredients into a sauté pan and scramble away. Quick and easy!

(*Side note*: please don't use non-stick pans for cooking: they're potentially toxic if scratched or overheated, and the compounds in them may be associated with elevated cholesterol levels in children.[2] What to use instead? Well, on the farm we have lovely cast-iron pans that I adore. I keep them rubbed down with a coating of olive oil, which over time produces a gorgeous, natural non-stick effect called seasoning.

Cast-iron cookware can actually boost your healthy iron intake,[3] rather than producing noxious fumes for your family to breathe, as non-stick pans can do if overheated. Plus, they have a wonderful old-fashioned texture and feel. When making scrambled eggs, get your cast-iron pan very hot before adding a dribble of olive oil, and then your eggs and other ingredients – this will make washing-up easier.)

If you're worried that eggs might endanger your heart because of their high level of dietary cholesterol, you can relax: a 2016 study from the University of Eastern Finland shows that a relatively high intake of dietary cholesterol, or eating one egg per day, is not associated with an elevated risk of coronary heart disease. The study did not establish a link between dietary cholesterol, or eating eggs, with thickening of the common carotid artery walls, either.[4]

In fact, scientists believe that eggs may have further antioxidant properties than have already been discovered, and more health benefits than we know of.[5] So, rediscover the farmhouse joy of eating eggs – laid by happy free-range chickens, of course.

What about tryptophan supplements?

Tryptophan supplements were popular some years back, until people started dying from EMS, or eosinophilia myalgia syndrome. EMS is an incurable, debilitating and sometimes fatal flu-like neurological condition caused by the ingestion of L-tryptophan supplements.

These supplements came from a single source, so EMS may have been caused by some unidentified contamination. The American Food and Drug Administration (FDA) placed a ban on the sale of L-tryptophan supplements and the incidence of EMS declined rapidly. The ban was lifted in 2005, and few new cases have been reported.[6]

Many people today continue to take tryptophan supplements, and report benefits. However, a shadow lingers over the subject. Personally, I'd rather get my tryptophan directly from natural sources like kefir and other foods – and avoid any risk!

Feed your good bugs: eat a rainbow!

Your inner ecosystem is all about biodiversity. Researchers tested how gut microbiota influence mood, and they found that in stressed subjects, there was less diversity in the types of bacteria present in the gut.

The gut and bowels are a very complex ecology, or they should be. The less diverse that environment is, the greater the disruption to the body.[7] Elderly people who are in poor health often have a lower diversity of microorganisms in their microbiome.[8]

Monoculture is bad: in our fields, in the world around us and in the ecosystem inside our gut. We want more species – a thriving wealth of interdependent life forms. The strength of an ecosystem is dependent on the number of relationships between its members. When you start to knock life forms off the ecological ladder, that ladder becomes fragile and starts to fall apart. Remember the wolves in the Yellowstone National Park story? We need more life forms, not fewer!

This is why diets like the low FODMAP diet – in which certain carbohydrates are eliminated – although temporarily helpful for IBS, don't provide a long-term solution to the problem. The answer lies not in eliminating food groups, but in expanding the diversity of bacterial species in your microbiome, and then expanding the numbers and kinds of foods that you eat, in order to feed all those happy, thriving bugs!

At the UK's Taymount Clinic, which performs faecal transplants and helps clients improve and maintain a healthy gut, experts look for donors with healthy microbiomes who eat 50 different kinds of food per week. So that's the goal! How many different kinds of food do you eat in a given week?

If you've got into the habit of avoiding almost all foods, in order to alleviate the abdominal pain, bloating, constipation and diarrhoea of IBS, this is good news for you. You're going to be able to get a lot of foods back into your diet. Again, it's a slow process, but there is joyful light at the end of this tunnel.

Shop for food by colour

We're all creatures of habit, and it's easy to fall into a rut with our food choices. What I suggest to my clients who have backed themselves into a frightened, bland corner with their eating habits, is this: take yourself on a field trip to the supermarket and choose your foods as if you were a seven-year-old child on a fun day out.

Walk up and down the fruit and veg aisle, and *shop with your eyes*. See something purple that looks attractive? Throw it into the basket. Gorgeous yellow colour? In it goes. Make a deal with yourself that you'll treat yourself to any fruit or vegetable that you like the look of. Orange, red, purple, blue and super dark green – bee-yoo-tiful!

Let yourself get excited about the colours. If you don't know what it is, or don't know what to do with it, that's okay: those foods are what smoothies are for.

(*Side note:* blending a fruit or vegetable is fine, as long as the pulp remains with it. Although juicing – taking the pulp away from the juice – has its advocates, it should be avoided while following the Kefir Solution. You need to eat the pulp to slow down the rate at which the food is converted to glucose inside your system; otherwise the wash of insulin that results will destabilize your microbiome and upset all your precious gut bugs.)

Obviously, if you know that you're allergic to a foodstuff, avoid it, for now. Over time, taking kefir will bring down the level of allergic response, and before too long you may find yourself able to enjoy things that you never dreamed you could eat.[9]

There's solid science behind this madness: shopping by colour and using your eyes will help switch on your body intuition. Deep down, your body knows what it needs! Also, the different, intense colours of the fruits and vegetables are due to different phytonutrients, which act as powerful antioxidants. Here are some examples:

Blue

Anthocyanins, which are found in purple and bluish foods like red cabbages, blueberries, and pomegranates, help protect your DNA, reduce inflammation and provide a wide range of antioxidants that help ward off damage to our cells.

Red

Red fruits and vegetables, such as raspberries, tomatoes, guavas, watermelons, kidney beans, cherries, strawberries and beetroot, are likely to be rich in the antioxidants lycopene and anthocyanins.

Orange and yellow

Most orange and yellow fruits and vegetables are rich in beta carotene, which your body converts to vitamin A: a nutrient that not only improves night vision, but also helps keep your skin, teeth and bones healthy. They also contain folate, an antioxidant that prevents neural tube defects in unborn babies.

Green

Green vegetables are good for your eyes, bones and teeth, and their vitamin K content helps your blood to clot properly.

White

White fruits and vegetables, including apples, pears, bananas, cauliflower and cucumber, are high in dietary fibre – helping to protect you from raised cholesterol – and antioxidant-rich flavonoids such as quercetin, which is abundant in apples and pears. They may also lower your risk of stroke, according to a group of Dutch researchers who published a study with the American Heart Association in 2011.

Mix it up!

You have trillions of different bug species in your gut, and they all eat different things. You need to think about consuming a variety of foods, so there's something in your diet for all your bugs. Fruit and veggies contain a wide array of plant compounds and tiny amounts of trace nutrients, creating a synergistic effect in which the total benefit is far greater than the sum of its parts.

That's one reason why a varied diet of real food works better than swallowing antioxidant supplements: any supplement you take may not be the exact one your body needs at that moment. A bowl of salad contains more than vitamins and minerals: plant matter also includes remnants of the hormones that plants produce to control how they grow, age and manage water intake.

Recently, scientists have reported that our gut microbes and our human cells may respond to these hormones, and even produce similar molecules of their own. This makes sense: we have co-evolved with plants over time, so it's not surprising to find that plant hormones have an impact on human health![10]

So, offer your gut bugs a smorgasbord of choices, with tons of beautiful, brightly coloured fruit and veg. Food is truly medicine for your body. And it should be fun, too. Having variety and colour in your life is part of being human.

Feed your good bugs: eat resistant starch

In order to keep your gut bugs healthy, you actually need to eat foods that you *can't* digest. Sounds crazy, right? Meet 'resistant starch': a type of dietary fibre that isn't fully absorbed by the body. Resistant starch is a good thing for both our gut health and our immune system – and scientists have only recently figured out *how* good.

Basically, the idea is this: you eat food and during the body's digestive process, it gets broken down by the bugs inside your gut. If the food is pretty lightweight stuff, like processed or packaged products, it's *all* digested in your stomach and small intestine. This means there's nothing left over at the end to pass on to the large intestine, where many of our gut bugs live.

But food that contains resistant starch can't be fully broken down in your stomach and small intestine. This means there are leftovers for the bugs to eat. They happily munch on the resistant starch and ferment it into butyrate, a beneficial fatty acid.[11]

Butyrate is the Holy Grail of the gut because it has powerful anti-inflammatory effects. In order to make our immune system work properly, we absolutely must eat foods that cause our good gut bugs to produce butyrate. Which means we must eat resistant starch in order to feed those bugs. And at the moment, most of us are not eating enough.

Think of resistant starch as a compost or 'super fertilizer' that feeds your good gut bacteria: when they are flourishing, they grow like crazy, producing vitamins, regulating your hormones, excreting toxins, and creating healing compounds that keep your gut healthy and functioning properly.

When you eat processed foods that are high in sugar and saturated fat, you 'feed the wrong wolf'. Bad bugs and harmful yeasts inside your body love this kind of diet! They flourish, grow out of control and overload your system with toxins called lipopolysaccharides

(LPS) that subsequently trigger inflammation, insulin resistance, pre-diabetes and ultimately, weight gain.

Just spare a thought for our poor good gut bugs. First we zap them with antibiotics. Then we blast them with sugar. Then we starve them by denying them healthy leftovers of resistant starch. It's no wonder that a large percentage of the population in the industrialized world is suffering from IBS, depression and anxiety!

The benefits of resistant starch

As your gut heals – as it will do when you follow the Kefir Solution eating principles – your good bugs will increase and crowd out the bad ones, decreasing inflammation in the process. You'll be 'feeding the right wolf'. Here's a quick summary of what resistant starch can do for you:[12]

- Increase the production of butyrate in the gut.

- Promote the growth of good bugs in the gut, while keeping the bad bugs at bay.

- Kill off pre-cancerous cells in your gut.

- Reduce inflammation.

- Help reduce the symptoms of IBS.[13]

Resistant starch may also help reduce the colorectal cancer risk that's associated with eating red meat. So if you're increasing your levels of tryptophan by eating red meat, it's absolutely imperative that you eat foods containing resistant starch as well.[14]

Which foods contain resistant starch?

Okay, so we now know that we want resistant starch in our diet, but where do we find it? Here are some good natural sources:

- Bananas that are slightly green, and plantains

- Cooked and cooled new or sweet potatoes *(see note on page 118)*

- Wholegrains

- Legumes (lentils, peas, beans)

- Chicory and dandelion leaves

- Jerusalem artichokes

- Psyllium husk

According to a study conducted at the University of Illinois at Urbana-Champaign in the USA, legumes are particularly good sources of both dietary fibre and resistant starch. Black beans contain the highest amount of total dietary fibre (43 per cent), and 63 per cent of their total starch content is resistant starch that makes it to the large intestine.

Researchers have also found that cereal grains contain resistant starch, but they are lower in fibre than legumes. Rolled oats, for example, have 15 per cent resistant starch when they reach the large intestine – one of many reasons that oats are a great choice for breakfast.

George C. Fahey Jr, who led the University of Illinois at Urbana-Champaign study, said: 'Flours don't have much resistant starch, because they are processed so much. A lot of grain-based foods also don't have very much resistant starch. But if we eat grain-based materials that are not heavily processed, and legumes, which we usually eat after minimal cooking, we get a lot of resistant starch and a lot of fibre as colonic [large intestine] foods.'[15]

Note: resistant starch needs to be consumed at room temperature. Food containing it must be cooked then cooled: think potato salad made with cold boiled *new* potatoes.[16] New potatoes or sweet potatoes are a better choice than old white potatoes, because the latter have a high glycaemic index. More on this later.

An easy way to get resistant starch into your diet is to use potato starch. I keep a bag of this around and add two tablespoons of it to my gluten-free flour mix (see the pancake recipe in Chapter 11). Be careful not to use potato flour, which is different and is *not* recommended. You can also add potato starch to a glass of water or goat's milk, or blend it into a smoothie.

I recommend adding about two tablespoons of resistant starch to your diet each day: have one tablespoon of potato starch with your morning meal or smoothie, and one tablespoon of psyllium husk powder, mixed into warm water and left to soak for 30 minutes, along with your evening meal.

Psyllium husk creates a feeling of fullness, and helps regulate blood sugar, so it may help you to resist late-night snacks. Psyllium husk added to water is also a remedy for constipation, and helps with diarrhoea.[17] (You'll find more specific remedies for constipation and diarrhoea in Shann's medical teas section of Chapter 12.)

As you begin to add resistant starch to your diet, you may experience some detox symptoms. But as the good bugs crowd out the bad ones, these will lessen and eventually completely go away.

And of course, don't forget to drink your kefir every day – to put those good bugs in there to begin with. Because good bugs + resistant starch = a happy immune system!

Starve your bad bugs: avoid sugar

What's the only sweetener you should use while you're following the Kefir Solution? In my opinion, it's 100 per cent pure stevia.

Stevia is brilliant stuff: it's made from a plant, is low GI (*see below*), has zero calories and is safe for diabetics. Stevia is not actually a sweetener at all – it just stimulates the sweet taste buds on your tongue, so you have the sensation of sweetness.

Stevia has been used for centuries as a bio-sweetener and a traditional treatment for diabetics, and studies show it may actually improve blood sugar control.[18] Stevia also appears to have anti-cancer, anti-inflammatory, antioxidant and antibacterial properties. Researchers particularly recommend its health benefits for diabetic patients, those wishing to lose weight and children.[19]

The sugar folks fought long and hard to keep stevia out of the UK and off the shelves – and who can blame them? You would do the same, if faced with an alternative to your product that had zero calories and actual health benefits.

The sugar barons lost the fight, though, and had to adopt a 'if you can't beat 'em, join 'em' approach, so stevia can now be found in many shops. A word of advice though: check the label on a stevia product carefully *before* you buy it. Most of the stevia you'll find in the supermarket is layered onto a dextrose base to give it extra bulk – and dextrose is sugar! Naughty marketers…

Which kind of stevia is best?

What you want is 100 per cent pure stevia – make sure it states that on the label. It comes as crystals, drops and clickers, I like the crystals and the clickers (handy for coffee and tea), but I don't like the drops, as I find them fiddly and I'm generally in a hurry. But that's just personal preference: you might find they work really well for you.

I usually order stevia online, or get it from a health food store. The pure stuff is pricey – but as it's something like 30 times as sweet as sugar, one bag will do you for a long, long time!

The only downside to stevia that I've found is that it's hard to bake with. It has an odd, fluffy texture, unlike the lovely grainy quality that sugar gives a cake. If you find a good way to bake with it, please do let me know, and we'll go into business together!

There is a baking version of stevia that has erythritol added for bulk. Erythritol is a sugar alcohol that's made by fermenting glucose. Like stevia, it doesn't raise your blood sugar, so it's safe for your microbiome.

The advantage of erythritol is that it creates the same shiny effect in low-calorie chocolate, adds bulk to dairy products and improves the shelf life of baked goods. Stevia and erythritol work for home baking because they're both heat-stable substances. It's safe enough, but I'm still not crazy about the results.

For baking I prefer to sweeten the mixture with whole, blended fruit and vegetables, like bananas and carrots, medjool dates or dried fruit. Dried fruit tends to have a similar glycaemic index (*see below*) to its non-dried counterpart, so is safe to use sparingly as a natural sweetener. Because dried fruit still has its fibre, the sugar goes into your bloodstream more slowly.

Dried apples, apricots, peaches and plums are all nice to work with. If you need to increase sweetness levels, you can top up with stevia until it's sweet enough for your taste.

Note: pregnant or nursing women shouldn't use stevia: whole stevia leaves were traditionally used as a contraceptive by the Guarani Indians in Paraguay. Those on blood pressure or diabetes medication should check with their doctor before using stevia-based products, as they may interact with these medications. People allergic to ragweed may be allergic to stevia as well.

Just say 'no' to sugar

Now that we've talked about adding stevia to your diet, let's talk about something you need to let go of when following the Kefir Solution: sugar. Sorry to say this, but it's a real baddie. Quite simply, sugar kills the good bugs in your microbiome.

Professor Cynthia Kenyon of the University of California, one of the world's top researchers in the field of ageing, experimented with giving glucose to worms, and found that it shortened their lifespan. Killed them right off. She claims that if you could only see what she's seen, in terms of what sugar does to living organisms, you'd never eat sugar again. She doesn't.[20]

Understanding as you now do the interaction between sugar, gut bugs, mental health and dopamine, you'll be unsurprised to hear that studies have found that eating too much sugar may increase the long-term risk of mental health disorders.

Researchers found that men who consumed more than 67g (just over 2¼oz) of sugar daily, from sweetened foods and beverages, were much more likely to develop anxiety, depression and other common mental disorders after five years, compared with men with a lower daily sugar intake.[21]

Are we shocked? We are not.

Sugar is death to your microbiome. Just like pouring bleach into a river, it will kill off the good bacteria that the kefir is putting into your system and undo all the good you've done. If you want to resolve your IBS, depression and anxiety, just say 'no' to sugar.

What about other sweeteners?

Can you eat honey and other natural sweeteners while following the Kefir Solution? Well, honey is brilliant stuff, but I treat it as medicine. It's a natural antibiotic. Here on the farm, if anyone has a cough or a cold (a rare event these days!) we make a mixture of honey, lemon and ginger, and drink it down.

We also apply sterile dressings that have been infused with honey to wounds, in order to promote rapid healing and prevent infection. I used these honey dressings on Rich's wound when he had the MRSA infection, and I always keep a few spare in my farmhouse first-aid kit – they're brilliant.[22] Honey should not be mixed with kefir, though, because its naturally antibiotic action will kill off the good kefir probiotics that you're trying to get into your system.

We don't mess with manuka honey – apparently, three times more manuka honey is on the shelves than is actually produced in New

Zealand, so the chances are good that you're being overcharged for fake manuka![23]

When we need honey on the farm, we use heather honey – the type that most beekeepers choose to eat. It's a little more expensive than regular honey, but nowhere near as pricey as manuka! It's a mono-honey (made from only one plant) that's been shown to be just as antibacterially effective as manuka.[24]

Honey is very high on the glycaemic index (*see below*) – almost as high as pure glucose – so don't use it as an everyday sweetener. It will rock your microbiome. The same goes for maple syrup and agave syrup. Maple syrup is even higher on the glycaemic index than honey, so it's no good for your microbiome, either.

And please *do not* use agave syrup. Agave nectar is about 85 per cent fructose, which is much higher than plain sugar, and can contribute to insulin resistance when consumed in large amounts.

I don't hold with artificial sweeteners, so those are out. Big badness there, I believe! Xylitol – mmm, well, I do chew xylitol gum because it's been shown to promote dental health. But stevia is the only thing that goes onto my farmhouse kitchen table.

Starve your bad bugs: avoid processed food

In terms of food, it's a jungle out there – and not in a good, biodiverse kind of way. If you walk out into the world hungry, you'll fall: because everything that's quick, easy and readily available is heavily processed and pumped full of the things that you need to avoid while following the Kefir Solution for your IBS, depression and anxiety.

How bad are such processed foods for your microbiome? *Really bad.*

Tim Spector, a professor of genetic epidemiology at King's College, London, wanted to find out what would happen to someone's gut microbiome if they ate McDonald's food for 10 days straight. His son, Tom, agreed to do the experiment and throughout the period, sent stool samples to different laboratories.

The results were described as 'astounding'. After just 10 days of eating fast food, Tom's stool samples revealed that his gut microbes had been 'devastated': about 40 per cent of his bacterial species, amounting to more than 1,400 different types, had been lost. This was a severe loss of microbial diversity, and in so little time.[25]

Imagine what a microbiome could look like after years and years of eating this way! If you typically eat a lot of high-fat, high-sugar, highly processed foods, you're committing systematic 'bugacide' – slaughtering millions of innocent little beings whose lives are in your care.

Remember, from their point of view, you make the weather. You control the mouth. Whatever you put in there, they just have to deal with it, or not. So if you can't do it for yourself, do it for your poor gut bugs!

The key to resisting the temptation of harmful processed food is *preparation*. You're going to need to think ahead, be smart and stock up on the foods that feed your good bugs. Cook your own lunch (more on this later) and take it to work with you.

Just remember that, when it comes to food, the modern world is not your friend. You're going to have to design your own little microbiome Eden, and work hard to feed it. Your happy, grateful gut bugs will reward you with improved mood and smooth, pain-free digestion. In Chapter 10, you'll find tips to shift your diet from 'processed food' to 'real food', in order to help heal your IBS, depression and anxiety.

Starve your bad bugs: avoid high GI foods

As far as your microbiome is concerned, sugar isn't just the stuff that tastes sweet. Your entire system – all of the magic bugs that make up your body, your muscles, brain, heart and liver, and drive all of the trillions of cascading actions that occur every second in there – needs energy to work. And this energy comes from the food you eat.

The bugs in your gut digest your food by mixing it with fluids in your stomach. During this process, sugar and starches in the food are broken down into another type of sugar called glucose. The bugs in your stomach and small intestine absorb the glucose, and then release it into your bloodstream. Once in the bloodstream, glucose can be used immediately for energy, or stored up for later use.

But blood glucose (or blood sugar, as it's also called) on its own is not enough to make things work. You also need a hormone made by the pancreas called insulin, in order to use or store glucose for energy. Without insulin, glucose just loiters around in the bloodstream, catcalling and wasting time – good for nothing!

So clever, hardworking little cells called beta cells run a constant monitoring system on the amount of glucose in your bloodstream. They check your blood glucose level every few seconds, and sense when they need to speed up or slow down the amount of insulin they're making and releasing. These poor little guys are just trying to keep everything stable. And usually, we don't make it very easy for them.

Different foods do different things to our blood sugar levels. And most of the food we eat these days dumps huge amounts of blood sugar into our system, all at once.

The glycaemic index

The glycaemic index (GI) rates various foods on the basis of how quickly they raise blood sugar levels. A low GI rating means that the food raises blood sugar levels a little, while a high GI rating means that the food raises it a lot, *all at once*. The glycaemic index compares everything to pure glucose.

To understand why this matters so much, imagine that you're making a fire in a fireplace using only newspaper. What's going to happen when you light it? The paper will flare up with a huge, bright whooooosh, and then fade right down before dropping flat. That's what happens inside your system when you eat something that has a high GI rating.

When we eat foods that have a high GI rating, the glucose level in the blood soars, and the beta cells trigger the pancreas to release a lot more insulin into the bloodstream, to deal with all the blood sugar. Then the excess insulin in our system causes us to crave more sugar. So we eat more sugar, the beta cells dump in more insulin – and *voila*, after enough cycles like this, we end up with Type 2 diabetes. Basically, we've exhausted our body's insulin system by causing repeated blood sugar spikes.

But here's the kicker: it's not just things that taste sweet that create this cycle. It's also anything that raises our blood sugar rapidly, and that includes everyday foods like potatoes and rice. The body burns these up super fast, like newspaper in a fireplace.

In order to work, your microbiome needs to be in 'homeostasis'. Remember that word from biology class? It means 'maintaining a constant internal environment'. This is what your poor hardworking system is trying to do. Dump a bunch of sugar in there, cause a quick, brief and hot 'paper' fire that soon dies down, and there's no way it can maintain a steady environment.

Sorry to be the bearer of bad news here, but old white potatoes turn to sugar in your system faster than ice cream. Same for both white and wholewheat bread: there's no difference in the rate that your body burns these two foods. (I know, seems so wrong!)

GI ratings for common foods

The glycaemic index compares everything to pure glucose, which has a rating of 100. Any food with a GI value over 70 is considered high; 56–69 is medium; and 55 or less is low. This chart shows the GI values of some everyday foods:

Food	Glycaemic index (glucose = 100)
White rice	86
Brown rice	66
White bread, average	71
Wholewheat bread, average	44
Pasta (white durum wheat spaghetti)	44
Old white potato (boiled)	82

Food	Glycaemic index (glucose = 100)
Sweet potato (boiled)	46
New potato (boiled)	62
Ice cream	57
Lentils	29
Chickpeas	10
Hummus	6
Oatmeal (steel-cut)	55

So, if eating foods with a high GI rating, like bread, rice and potatoes, is like burning newspaper in our system, causing a big rush of blood sugar and destabilizing our microbiome, what the heck are we supposed to eat to help our good bugs?

Choose slow-burning foods

What we want to do is build our fire with wood, not newspaper. We're after foods that will burn slowly inside our system, keeping it ticking over, and blood sugar trickling steadily into it over time. It's the abrupt surges in sugar – the big newspaper flares – that upset our body and disrupt our microbiome.

Think foods high in fibre that take longer to digest and therefore produce a slower rise in blood sugar levels. Think oatmeal. Think pulses. Anything you have to chew a lot! Low GI grains like amaranth, millet, buckwheat and quinoa are good. Protein is good.

Think eggs, grass-fed cheese and butter. 'Good' fats found in foods such as avocados, nuts, seeds, oily fish, olive oil and flaxseed oil are helpful. Pasta, surprisingly, is pretty low GI! It has to do with the physical organization of the starch granules in the pasta dough. But cook pasta al dente, and don't overconsume it.

Love potatoes? Choose sweet potatoes – although it seems as if 'sweet' would translate to higher blood sugar, it doesn't! New potatoes sneak in at 62, beating a boiled white potato at 82. The good news is that a new potato salad made the day before, tossed with a vinaigrette dressing and kept in the fridge, will have a much lower GI rating than old white potatoes served steaming hot from the pot.

There are a couple of simple reasons for this. The cold storage increases the potatoes' resistant starch content by more than a third and the acid in the vinaigrette – whether it's made with lemon/lime juice or vinegar – will slow down the process.

One food that we often think of as healthy is commercial fruit juice. Fruit juice, which has the pulp removed, burns in your system very quickly. So don't juice your fruit: blend it instead! Whizz up a whole piece of fruit in a bullet blender and drink it with the pulp included – it will burn inside your system much more slowly.

So, what does all this have to do with your IBS, anxiety and depression? Everything! Remember: too much sugar kills off the good bugs in your microbiome that make the serotonin you need. And that means too much systemic blood sugar, not just the sweet white stuff.

Destabilize your microbiome, and the results will show up both in your gut and your brain. You want to eat things that will slowly trickle blood sugar into your system, keeping your microbiome platform steady and secure. And avoid things that wobble your microbiome platform, causing general panic and upheaval inside your system!

Don't irritate your gut: avoid cow dairy

If you're struggling with IBS, depression or anxiety, you may well be allergic to cow's milk. Cow's milk is the number one allergy among children and this can persist throughout adulthood.

Until recently, scientists believed that cow's milk allergy was relatively rare in adults, especially when there were no symptoms suggestive of food allergy. But a recent article in *Allergy and Asthma Proceedings* reported that in a study, more than half of the adult patients with presumed 'milk intolerance' weren't just intolerant, but actually allergic to cow's milk, as shown by an allergy skin test.

Forty-three per cent of the study participants had allergy symptoms that involved the skin (hives, eczema) and the nasal passages or lungs (asthma), as well as stomach complaints.[26] This means that many more adults are allergic to cow's milk than was previously believed.

So what's the big problem with cow's milk? Most people who are allergic to cow's milk are actually reacting to A1 casein, which is a protein found in cow's milk. A1 casein is highly inflammatory in some people, and inflammation is at the root of most diseases.

A1 casein can contribute to gastrointestinal issues, including IBS, Crohn's disease, leaky gut and ulcerative colitis, as well as autoimmune skin conditions such as eczema, psoriasis, rosacea and acne. The most frequent symptoms among the common manifestations of cow's milk allergy are gastrointestinal.[27]

There are some cows that don't produce A1 casein, like Jersey and Guernsey cows. But most cows in the USA, Western Europe and Australia are Holstein and Friesian, which are A1 casein producers.

Cow's milk also contains more than 20 other allergens that can cause allergic reactions. These symptoms – which are often confused with seasonal allergy symptoms – can range from hives and runny noses to abdominal cramping and colic in babies.

In his book *Don't Drink Your Milk!* Frank Oski, former paediatrics director at Johns Hopkins University School of Medicine, Maryland, estimated that half of all iron deficiency in US infants results from cow's milk-induced intestinal bleeding. This is a staggering number, given than 15 per cent of American under-twos suffer from iron-deficiency anaemia.

The infants, it seems, drink so much milk (which is very low in iron) that they have little appetite left for foods containing iron; at the same time, the milk, by inducing gastrointestinal bleeding, causes iron loss.

Choose goat dairy

So what can you drink instead of cow's milk? Goat's milk!

Goat's milk contains only A2 casein, which produces none of the inflammatory effects of A1 casein. Protein-wise, goat's milk is the closest milk to human breast milk. One study suggested that goat's milk, when used as the first protein after breastfeeding, is less allergenic for babies than cow's milk.[28]

Goat's milk is also easier to digest than cow's, high in calcium, low in cholesterol, helps to address iron and magnesium deficiency, improves the skin, and is a safe and natural way to treat osteoporosis. In the Western world, we tend to overlook goat's milk in favour of cow's, which is a shame because goat's milk is nutritious, healthy, and fabulous for both skin and gut.

In fact, after conducting a study into the nutritional characteristics of goat's milk, researchers at the University of Granada in Spain declared it a 'natural functional food': that's something that delivers additional or enhanced health benefits beyond its basic nutritional value.

They also found that goat's milk has more oligosaccharides, with a composition similar to that of human milk. These compounds reach the large intestine undigested and act as prebiotics (substances that make the pre-existing bugs in your gut healthier, so they can out-compete the bad bugs).

Goat's milk has a lower proportion of lactose (milk sugar) than cow's milk, which makes it easier to digest; many people with lactose intolerance can easily tolerate goat's milk. Goat's milk also has smaller fat molecules than cow's milk and a healthier type of fat: goat's milk has 30–35 per cent medium-chain fatty acids, while cow's has only 15–20 per cent. These fatty acids are a quick source of energy and aren't stored as body fat.[29]

Goat's milk fat reduces total cholesterol levels and maintains adequate levels of triglycerides and transaminases (GOT and GPT), which makes it helpful for the prevention of heart disease.[30]

Goat's milk is rich in calcium and phosphorus in a bioavailable form, which helps with bone formation. It also has more zinc and selenium than cow's milk: these essential micronutrients also help prevent neurodegenerative diseases.

For all these reasons, the Spanish scientists concluded that 'the consumption [of goat's milk] should be promoted among the population in general, especially among those with allergy or intolerance to cow's milk, malabsorption, high cholesterol levels, anaemia, osteoporosis or prolonged treatments with iron supplements.'[31]

It's relatively easy these days to find goat's milk, cheese, butter and yogurt in any quality supermarket. So switch over to goat dairy, and remove cow dairy from your diet for good.

Don't irritate your gut: choose 'good grains'

What's a 'good grain'? Let's start by examining what's *not* a good grain: in a word, *wheat*. Unfortunately, wheat is a 'bad grain'. Why? Because it contains a protein called gluten, which is a nasty allergen that triggers IBS, anxiety and depression.

The problem is that in Western Europe, we're absolutely addicted to wheat, and food manufacturers put it into almost everything we eat! Other cultures do a better job than us on this count, and tend to consume many different kinds of grain.

For example, the Russians eat buckwheat for breakfast and call it kasha, and the Japanese make their soba noodles out of it. Amaranth is consumed regularly in Africa, Indonesia, China and India, but few people in the UK have even heard of it!

We've taken one grain that's not very good for us – wheat – and now use it almost exclusively in our food products. We're going to have to push those grain boundaries out a bit, and adopt some better grain choices from our neighbours around the world.

How about barley and rye? Barley is low GI, and has many health benefits in terms of blood sugar. However, it does contain gluten, so it should be avoided while you're following the Kefir Solution. Rye bread has a lower GI than white or wholewheat bread, but it also contains gluten, so I suggest you avoid it as well.

However, I do *not* recommend that you avoid grains altogether. Wholegrains are a good source of nutrients, fibre and vitamins, and they also make you feel full and content after eating. So they're important!

The trick is to choose your 'good grains' carefully. What you want here is grains that are both low GI *and* gluten-free, so that they will:

1. Burn slowly inside your system, trickling sugar gently into the microbiome.

2. Refrain from irritating your gut, so that it can heal.

Here are some low GI, gluten-free alternatives to wheat that are helpful for healing your gut. In Chapter 11, you'll find cooking instructions and ideas for using them as a base for your meals.

Oatmeal

This is the old classic, but it's as good as food gets, being both low GI and anti-inflammatory. A bowl of porridge is the perfect breakfast, especially if you add a spoonful of coconut oil and a handful of blueberries.

Oatmeal is naturally gluten-free, but if you have coeliac disease it's worth paying extra for oatmeal labelled as gluten-free, as this means it's been grown in an exclusion zone where no bird can drop a seed of anything other than oats, thus avoiding gluten contamination.

Buckwheat

Despite its name, this nutty-tasting beauty is unrelated to wheat and contains no gluten. Buckwheat isn't actually a grain, either: it's a seed that's high in protein and fibre. It's good for digestive disorders, supports heart health and can help prevent diabetes.

In fact, buckwheat seeds, also called 'groats', are so nutrient and antioxidant dense that they're often called a 'superfood'. You can use sweet or savoury toppings for dishes containing buckwheat.

Amaranth

Amaranth is a native crop of Peru, and it's grown throughout the rest of South America too, as well as North America, Africa, India, China and Russia. This grain is becoming increasingly popular today because of its startling health benefits. As well as being a great source of protein, it reduces inflammation, improves bone health, lowers cholesterol, fights diabetes, aids digestive health and promotes weight loss.

Quinoa

Quinoa (pronounced *keen*-wah) originated in the mountainous regions of South America some 7,000 years ago. This grain has gained popularity in the last few years because of its significant health benefits as a nutritious 'superfood'. High in protein and a great source of fibre, it's also an antioxidant that supports heart health. It also helps prevent cancer and diabetes, and fights disease.

Quinoa is very plain-tasting, and is therefore highly versatile as an ingredient.

Millet

If you think millet sounds like bird food, you're not alone! While widely referred to as a grain, millet is actually a seed. And while birds do love it, it's easy to see why humans choose it, too. Millet is high in fibre and is also an alkaline food, meaning it's easily digestible and is a good option for those with a sensitive stomach.

If you've never cooked with millet, you'll be pleasantly surprised. Depending on the recipe, millet can have a creamy texture like mashed potatoes, or a fluffier, slightly crunchy one like quinoa or rice.

Sorghum

It's still hard to find 100 per cent wholegrain sorghum grains in most stores, but you can often find sorghum ground into a fine flour that can be used in various ways for cooking and baking. It's a common ingredient in gluten-free flour blends, which are convenient, healthy and perfect for baking and other uses. Sorghum flour is white or beige in colour and has a mild taste, making it a useful wheat substitute.

Gram flour

Gram flour (also called chickpea flour) is made from ground chickpeas, and it's surprisingly tasty! If your only contact with chickpeas has been adding them to a salad or occasionally eating hummus, then you're missing out on some of the serious benefits of gram flour. High in fibre and protein, gram flour is also very filling, so it's definitely worth trying out as an alternative to wheat flour.

Don't irritate your gut: limit lectins

Nothing wants to be eaten, including plants. Like anything else out there, plants want to survive until they get to germinate and reproduce. So, over time, they have developed a clever 'don't-eat-me' mechanism called lectins.

Lectins are sugar-binding plant proteins that attach to cell membranes and create pain inside the digestive system of the animal eating the bean or seed: to discourage that animal in future. For our purposes, you can think of lectins as toxins that will cause inflammation inside the gut – something you really need to avoid when you're trying to heal IBS, depression and anxiety!

Can you go entirely lectin-free? Not really. Doing so would eliminate most plant foods, which should ideally make up a large proportion of your diet. Instead, I suggest you avoid the nastiest lectins, and deal with the others through proper food preparation and cooking.

One of the main offenders is wheatgerm agglutinin, or WGA. On the lectin spectrum, WGA is even worse than gluten! So this means that bread is right out, especially wholewheat bread, which in terms of lectin content is even worse than white bread. If you still choose to eat bread, try sourdough (even though it's still high GI): it's made by a process of fermentation, which helps break down the lectins.

The following lectin-rich foods are best avoided:

- Corn (maize) in all its forms: cornmeal, corn oil, sweetcorn, popcorn. Corn is so high in lectins that 'corn gluten meal' is used as a natural herbicide. Corn pops up in a lot of places you wouldn't expect it: baked goods, condiments, sauces and salad dressings.

- Casein A1 milk – i.e. standard cow's milk that you buy from the shops. As we've previously discussed, milk from sheep, goats and some Jersey cows is fine, because it contains Casein A2, not the problematic A1. A1 is metabolized in your gut to make beta-casomorphin, which can attach to the beta cell of your pancreas and incite an autoimmune attack.

- Peanuts, cashews and *unfermented* soya bean/soybean products. If you want to eat soya, make sure it's traditionally fermented.

- Members of the nightshade family: tomatoes, old white potatoes (*see information about preparation on page 141*), aubergine/eggplant, peppers/bell peppers and goji berries

Reducing or removing lectins from food

If you're choosing foods like dried beans, pulses, seeds or grains – which I hope you are, for the resistant starch they contain – you need to sprout, soak or cook them correctly before eating them, because they are high in lectins.

Get into the habit of soaking dried beans overnight before cooking them, or try sprouting them (*see instructions for both below*). Grains can be cooked or sprouted and seeds can be sprouted, too. It's a bit of an adjustment, preparing these foods in this way, but it ain't rocket science, and you can do it. If cooking these foodstuffs, remember to let them cool to room temperature before eating them, in order to maximize their resistant starch.

Lentils are a pulse, and most recipes say that you don't have to soak them before cooking. However, in order to break down the lectins they contain, and make them easy on your digestive system, I do recommend soaking lentils overnight in plenty of cold water. Add one tablespoon of apple cider vinegar or lemon juice, to help the lectin breakdown process.

Plant lectins are most effectively neutralized when foods are cooked in a pressure cooker, so this handy kitchen gadget may be a worthwhile investment.

Sprout your own

Getting a sprouter to germinate dried beans, seeds, grains or pulses will enable you to produce a constant supply of delicious microgreens for you and your family, in any season. It's well worth the small investment and the effort involved to create this new habit in the kitchen.

Sprouted microgreens are fresh, healthy, relatively inexpensive and free from any chemicals. And you can't buy them from the shops because they rarely sell anything besides mustard or watercress. Microgreens will give you the nutrient boost that you can't get from the iceberg lettuce that we so often see on the supermarket shelves here in the UK!

A GUIDE TO SPROUTING

Here's what you need to get started:

A sprouter: this is simply a jar with a lid through which you can strain water. Or you could just use a rubber band and some cheesecloth over the top of a clean jar.

Any wholegrain, bean, seed or pulse. Broccoli seeds are great as they have powerful health benefits, or you can try beet, bok choy, radish and alfalfa. Make sure that the seeds or grains you sprout are organic and not coated with chemicals (as those from commercial plant nurseries sometimes are).

INSTRUCTIONS

- ✤ Put your chosen seeds, beans, pulses or grains in your sprouter or jar. Don't overfill it – shoot for about one-third full – as at the next stage, the contents may expand to up to three times their size.

- ✤ Cover the seeds/beans/pulses/grains with water, up to around 5cm (2 in) below the lip of the sprouter/jar. Attach the mesh lid that came with your sprouter, or the cheesecloth/rubber band on your jar – *don't use an airtight lid.*

- ✤ Soak overnight. In the morning, drain the water out of the sprouter/ jar, replace the cloth and let the sprouter/jar sit on the kitchen worktop, out of direct sunlight.

- ✤ Every 12 hours, add water to the sprouter/jar, swish it around and then drain it out again. After about 24–36 hours, you'll start seeing little white tails as the sprouting process begins. Depending on how many items you're sprouting and the room conditions (heat, etc), this process could take up to four days.

✦ You can eat your sprouts any time after you start to see the little tails emerge. When they are ready, tip them onto a double layer of paper towels and leave them to dry out a bit. Then store them in an airtight container in the fridge.

✦ You can add your sprouts to salads, soups or smoothies, or just eat a handful for a gut-healthy snack!

Preparing and cooking dried beans

Beans are great, but if you're using dried beans, rather than canned, you need to prepare and cook them properly to reduce their lectin content. Never eat raw or undercooked beans, as they can have acute, toxic effects. As few as five beans can cause a reaction reminiscent of food poisoning, so to make beans safe to eat, be sure to do the following:

• Soak the beans in water for at least 12 hours before cooking, changing the water at least once. Adding baking soda to the soaking water will boost the neutralization of lectins even further.

• Discard the soaking water and rinse the beans. Cook for at least 15 minutes on a high heat. Cooking beans on too low a heat can actually increase toxicity levels by up to five times or more.

Cooking potatoes for gut health

The lectin content in potatoes will also be reduced by cooking, although these lectins tend to be more resistant to heat than those in beans. Cooking potatoes will reduce their lectin content by 50 to 60 per cent. Remember to cool them afterwards, to increase the amount of resistant starch they contain

The Kefir Solution eating principles in a nutshell

Here's a summary of the programme's eating principles:

1. Feed the good bugs by:

- Eating protein-rich foods that are high in tryptophan – including kefir, nuts, eggs, seeds, beans, poultry, fish, yogurt, cheese and 70 per cent or more cocoa solids chocolate.

- Eating a rainbow of fruit and vegetables.

- Eating resistant starch.

2. Starve the bad bugs by:

- Avoiding sugar (use 100 per cent pure stevia instead).

- Avoiding processed food (eat real food instead).

- Avoiding high GI foods (eat low GI foods instead).

3. Prevent gut irritation by:

- Avoiding cow dairy (eat goat dairy instead).

- Avoiding gluten (eat gluten-free 'good grains' instead).

- Reducing plant lectins (by cooking, sprouting and soaking foods).

THE KEFIR SOLUTION SUCCESS STORY

*My IBS dated from 2004, when I split from my husband. We had
a substantial house and garden, and worry over finances, holding
down my job and stress in general seemed to be the trigger for it.*

*I went to my doctor and was referred for a colonoscopy, and I tried
all the over-the-counter medications. I tried apple cider vinegar and
activated charcoal, too – you name it, I tried it! Nothing worked.*

*It made me so miserable! I had a quarter-acre vegetable plot and
was very competitive in the village show, but it got to the point
where I couldn't tolerate eating any of my homegrown vegetables.
I couldn't eat anything without feeling uncomfortable.*

*I had awful problems with urinary tract infections, which were
exacerbated by three doses of antibiotics. My gut was in disarray. It
was so depressing: not severely, but it did make me feel down.*

*I stumbled across Chuckling Goat after searching and searching for
answers on the Internet. I read through the anecdotal reviews, and
then decided to order the kefir. Once I started taking it, I got back
my positive outlook on life. My mood improved, and I had more
energy. I wasn't walking around feeling totally fed up.*

*Halfway through my second lot of kefir, about six weeks in, I
started to improve quite quickly. I was able to eat everything – any
fruits and vegetables – without ill effects. I remember thinking,* Oh
my God, everything is going to be fine.

*I had a friend with severe acid reflux, and the doctor gave him
medicine for it. He couldn't tolerate it: it was so bad that he had to
sleep upright. I recommended kefir to his wife, and he's been taking
it for a while. He can now sleep normally, and his acid reflux is
fine. I've recommended kefir to several other friends as well.*

Now everything is good. No more lying awake all night! The IBS has been very good now for six months. I've made no other changes. I can tolerate everything! When I received the first lot of kefir I followed the instructions, and steered away from everything I was supposed to. Now I just eat whatever I feel like having! I'm so delighted to have found kefir: it's changed my life.

ANNETTE BLACKWELL, 64, RETIRED TEACHER, HAMPSHIRE, UK

Chapter 11

The Kefir Solution
Eating Plan

So, how do the Kefir Solution eating principles I outlined in the last chapter translate into real life? On the farm, we're always super busy, so all of our meals are streamlined, and quick and easy to prepare. I like to think in terms of efficient delivery systems: I'm trying to get as many beneficial nutrients as possible into both myself, and two resistant males!

The following is how I handle the food issue in a typical day at Chuckling Goat. I suggest that you follow this format strictly for nine weeks, to get accustomed to the new way of eating, and then take off and allow yourself a bit of freestyle.

- **Breakfast**: overnight kefir oats

- **Snacks**: gluten-free pancakes, nuts, dried coconut flakes, fruit

- **Lunch**: an ugly food bowl (caught your attention there, didn't I? It will all make sense very soon!)

- **Supper**: a meat or fish dish or a soup, with vegetables and grain on the side

- **Treats**: coffee, 70 per cent cocoa solids dark chocolate

Sounds simple, right? Let's break it down into more detail:

Breakfast

Overnight kefir oats is my go-to breakfast. It ticks all my boxes: fast, tasty, low GI, gluten-free, satisfying, superfood-charged, rich in resistant starch and a boost to the nervous system. What's not to like?

Note: you can use your daily 170ml/6fl oz dose of goat's milk kefir in this recipe. The oats won't prevent the kefir from adhering to the wall of the gut, so it's fine to consume it in this way.

Overnight kefir oats
Serves 1

170ml/6fl oz goat's milk kefir

A handful of organic jumbo oats

60g/2oz fruit of your choice

1 tbsp chia seeds

100 per cent pure stevia, to taste

Optional extras: pinch of sea salt, ½ tsp natural vanilla extract

Method

1. The night before, soak the oats and the chia seeds in the kefir.

2. When you're ready to drink the oat/kefir mixture the following morning, add the fruit and the optional extras. Place in a high-

powered blender and whizz until smooth. Sweeten with stevia if desired.

The ultimate breakfast

Overnight kefir oats is a real powerhouse, and it works in a variety of ways. First, leaving the oats in the kefir overnight means you're soaking a grain in an acidic mixture, which helps break down the phytic acid it contains: this is an 'anti-nutrient' that interferes with digestive enzymes and inhibits the absorption of minerals.

Cooking is one way to break down phytic acid in foods that contain it, but research suggests that soaking them in something acidic may be even better at improving their digestibility.

Why soak the chia seeds?

You may have heard about the health benefits of chia seeds; they *are* great, but they need to be soaked *before* eating, and this recipe provides an easy way to do that. Chia have a mucilaginous shell coating, and will absorb up to 12 times their weight in water – and you don't want them doing that inside your throat!

Like all other seeds, chia seeds contain phytic acid, which prevents birds from eating them. Soaking the chia in the acidic kefir will activate the seed, making it more bio-available to your body and helping prevent blood sugar spikes; it will also decrease cholesterol and keep you hydrated for longer. Hydrated chia seeds also slow digestion: it takes longer for your stomach to empty, so you feel full for longer.

So, you're soaking the oats and the chia seeds in the kefir overnight. You need to wait until morning to add the fruit, though, because the fructose (fruit sugar) it contains will degrade the probiotics if it sits with them overnight.

This is why you need to source unflavoured kefir – any fruit or other sweeteners added during the production process will kill the good bugs as it sits on the shelf! Keep your kefir pure, and only add fruit and/or stevia right before you're ready to drink it.

Why raw oats and not cooked?

Raw oats are one of the very best sources of resistant starch. Remember, resistant starch is what's left over after certain foods are digested; these leftovers are what your gut bugs eat. This is one of the reasons why a diet high in processed foods is so bad for you – your body burns right through that lightweight stuff and there's nothing left for your friendly gut bugs to eat. Gut bugs eat resistant starch and happily produce butyrate, so gut bugs love raw, soaked oatmeal!

Oats are also one of the best remedies for stress. In traditional herbal medicine, oats are specifically recommended for helping with nervous disability and exhaustion, especially when associated with depression. Oats are used as a nerve tonic, both relaxant and stimulatory, to strengthen the entire nervous system.

As a side benefit, oatmeal boosts weight loss. It's digested slowly, triggering the release of digestive acids shown to suppress the appetite and speed up calorie burning. According to one study, swapping just 5 per cent of our daily carbohydrates for foods containing resistant starch could boost our metabolism by 23 per cent.

The outer layers of oats contain a form of fibre called oat beta-glucan, and at least 3 grams of this daily has been shown to reduce cholesterol levels by 5 to 10 per cent.[1] You'd need to eat two servings of regular oatmeal daily to reap the benefits. But just one bowl of overnight kefir oats may be equally, if not more, effective.

Overnight kefir oats also has a creamy, pudding-like consistency that makes it pleasant to eat – it definitely has the yummm factor! That's important because if you enjoy something, you may be more likely to absorb more nutrients from it.

In a joint study, researchers from Sweden and Thailand found that Thai women fed a traditional Thai dish absorbed twice as much iron than a group of Swedish women who ate the same meal, which they reported not enjoying. And when the two groups ate traditional Swedish fare, the Swedes absorbed 50 per cent more iron than the Thai women who didn't care for the meal.[2]

So, the more enjoyable your overnight kefir oats experience, the more zinc, copper, magnesium, biotin and B vitamins you may absorb.

Other ideas for overnight kefir oats

Here are some daily variations on the basic overnight kefir oats recipe (*see page 146*); all recipes serve one. Use these ideas to vary the fruit/seed part of the recipe.

Sunday: exotic holiday
60g/2oz mango; 60g/2oz pineapple; 1 tbsp coconut oil

Monday: blueberry surprise
60g/2oz blueberries

Tuesday: bounty bliss
1 tsp coconut oil; 1 tsp raw cacao powder

Wednesday: banana boat
1 banana; 1 tbsp almond butter

Thursday: carrot cake
Half a large carrot, peeled and cut into chunks; ½ tsp cinnamon

Friday: pina colada
60g/2oz pineapple; half a banana; 1 tsp coconut oil

Saturday: strawberry slushy
60g/2oz fresh strawberries; ½ tsp pure vanilla extract

Snacks

For a quick snack, I keep a selection of nuts around. In a US study, scientists found a link between eating nuts and higher levels of serotonin. It took only 30g/1oz of mixed nuts (raw, unpeeled walnuts, almonds and hazelnuts) a day to produce these beneficial effects.[3]

In a Spanish study, patients given a nut-rich diet produced a higher level of metabolites derived from the metabolism of tryptophan and serotonin, fatty acids and polyphenols. This gives more weight to the hypothesis that these molecules could be at the root of certain health benefits observed in other studies.[4]

I also love to keep a bowl of unsweetened dried coconut flakes around: they release a lovely little rush of coconut oil when you bite down on them, and they contain fibre. Fruit also makes a great snack, especially with a square of goat's cheese. Bananas are particularly good – full of tryptophan, as you know.

No bread? No problem!

Regular bread containing gluten is not recommended while following the Kefir Solution. But we all miss it! It's not just the convenience of using it as a base onto which we can layer things: we're just used to having bread by the side of our plates, to fill us up and add texture and fibre to a meal. So here are two gluten-free options that you can have instead. Meet the pancake and kefir soda bread.

Pancakes are vastly underrated in the UK, where they are mostly relegated to a once-a-year outing and covered with sugar. In the USA, pancakes are eaten more often, but they are ring-fenced for breakfast and smothered in high GI maple syrup.

So, I officially encourage you to reboot your ideas about pancakes. A pancake is a simple flat bread cooked in a griddle or a frying pan, and nothing could be faster, easier or more tempting!

We fry up a stack of the following 'save-my-snacktime' babies every three days or so, wrap them in clingfilm and put them in the fridge (where they'll keep for up to four days). For a snack, or lunch, you can then pop them in the toaster to make them warm and crispy. These pancakes can be sweet or savoury – serve them with the topping of your choice from the suggestions below.

Save-my-snacktime pancakes

Makes 8 pancakes

500ml/17fl oz kefir

200ml/7fl oz goat's milk

1 free-range egg

250g/8oz gram flour (chickpea flour)

200g/7oz other gluten-free flour: choose either buckwheat, quinoa, sorghum, millet flakes or coconut flour

1 tbsp potato starch (not potato flour)

1 tsp bicarbonate of soda

½ tsp sea salt

Goat's butter or coconut oil

Method

1. Combine the kefir, egg and goat's milk in a bowl.

2. In another bowl, mix the flours, bicarbonate of soda and salt.

3. Melt 1 tbsp of the goat's butter and pour onto the dry ingredients.

4. Slowly incorporate the flour mixture into the kefir mixture to produce a batter. (Make sure the batter is not thin and soupy, otherwise you'll get crepes. It should be a nice firm batter that is pourable. If it's too thin, add more flour.)

5. Heat a griddle or frying pan to a medium heat and add about 1 tbsp of goat's butter/coconut oil. Scoop the pancake batter with a ladle and pour into the pan.

6. Cook each pancake for a few minutes on each side. Flip them over when you see bubbles appear on the surface.

If you like a sweet pancake, add 100 per cent pure stevia to taste, or top it with fruit, such as blueberries or strawberries. If you prefer yours savoury, add butter, soft goat's cheese, hummus, guacamole or almond butter.

Kefir soda bread

This bread is hearty and crumbly. It's a bit challenging to make sandwiches with it, but it goes a treat alongside soups, stews and slow-cooked meals.

240ml/8fl oz kefir (milk or water kefir)

130g/4½oz organic buckwheat flour

70g/2¼oz organic quinoa flour or oat flour

70g/2¼oz organic almond flour/meal

30g/1oz soaked oat groats (optional)

½ tsp sea salt

1 tsp baking soda

Method

1. Place the buckwheat flour and the kefir in a glass bowl and mix to combine. Soak overnight, or for at least 12 hours.

2. Preheat the oven to 200°C/400°F/Gas 6.

3. Sieve the remaining dry ingredients into a glass bowl; then add the wet ingredients. Try to mix them as little as possible. Leave the dough in the bowl for 10 minutes.

4. Add a little flour to your hands. Put the dough (leave it in the shape it took on while in the bowl) on a baking sheet lined with a greased sheet of parchment paper. Dust the dough lightly with a little gluten-free flour and cut a deep cross in the top.

5. Bake for 30 minutes until brown on the outside.

Enjoy this warm, dripping with goat's butter!

Lunch

In our culture, we tend to use wheat products as a base for our lunch (and supper), on top of which we load stuff: bread makes a sandwich, pasta gets a sauce, pizza dough gets, well, pizza toppings. And as we discussed earlier, all of these foods contain gluten, which is going to irritate the lining of your gut.

The other things we often use as a base are baked potatoes and rice, both of which are bad choices because they have high GI ratings and burn too quickly inside our system – which means they harm our microbiome.

But what's a person to *eat* while following the Kefir Solution?! If you take the base away, it's difficult to know what to put things on. What's a sandwich without the bread? A baked potato without the potato?

Meet the food bowl

But don't despair, because I have a different concept for you, and it can be applied to both lunch and supper. Instead of thinking sandwich, pasta or rice… think *bowls* of food. You're going to create a delicious bowl of food using a good grain as a base. Then on top of that good grain, you're going to layer any meat/vegetable or sauce combination that you fancy, as long as it's in line with the Kefir Solution eating principles.

Why a bowl? Well, the good grains we're going to switch to – amaranth, millet, quinoa, buckwheat and oatmeal – don't stick together into a base, so we need a bowl to contain them. Part of the reason they don't stick together is that they don't contain gluten – gluten is the sticky protein in wheat that makes it stick together. But we're going to use a bowl to hold our food instead.

Rock your ugly!

Is your lunch ugly enough? This is an important question, because food bowls can be *ugly*. We're used to sandwiches, which are contained and non-messy. But the healthy ingredients you're combining in your food bowl can be messy.

There's a certain beauty here too, and I know you're going to find it! But it's important to *own* the ugly. If you create a bowl-to-go for work or school (also known as a Tupperware container) – suggestions for these coming up – you should flaunt its healthy ugliness with pride!

The principle behind the food bowl is to combine three elements: *base, topping, sauce.* Just use the following calculator to make your own creations!

Food bowl base

This can be a good grain or a noodle made from a good grain – think quinoa, millet, amaranth, sorghum, oats, buckwheat.

What makes this work is that good grains are just grains: they're neither savoury nor sweet, and they don't have much taste on their own. Their job in the food bowl is to fill you up, reduce inflammation inside the system, and provide the fibre that your gut bugs both need and love.

So they're a base for you to work with – the dressmaker's dummy, so to speak, on top of which you're going to design a variety of fabulous outfits.

Food bowl topping

On top of your good grain base, add a protein food (fish, meat, eggs, cheese), vegetables or fruit, and a nut/seed/bean/pulse of your choice. You can vary the quantities according to your taste. Here are some suggestions for each element:

Protein: salmon, sardines, chicken breast, turkey breast, lamb, beef, pork; dairy: eggs, goat's yogurt, goat's cheese.

Vegetables/fruit: choosing three types will fill your bowl with colour, texture and nutrients – all goodies for your gut bugs! Add more leafy greens if desired.

Think seasonally: spring combinations might be asparagus, radish and baby carrots. Summertime is perfect for spinach, cucumber and anything else just picked. Autumn is great for Brussels sprouts, sweet potato, squash and kale. Winter is a good time to use root vegetables like turnips, parsnips and beets, which can be complemented with immune-boosting ginger and turmeric.

If you're thinking breakfast, the world is your fruit bowl! Apples, pears, berries, cherries, pineapple, mango, unsweetened coconut flakes, oranges, tangerines, the list goes on – pick things you like, things you know you're not allergic to. Bananas are particularly brilliant because they're mild, creamy and contain high levels of tryptophan.

Time-saving hack: in a perfect world we would all be growing our own chemical-free veg and getting our hands into the soil (more on this topic later). But in the real world, we don't all have the luxury of growing our own, and life is busy!

So if you're tight on time, go for salad bar vegetables from your local supermarket, pre-cut bagged veggies or frozen vegetables. Don't get hung up on perfection. Any improvement is better than no improvement – let's keep it real!

Nuts/seeds/beans/pulses: try almonds, pistachios, walnuts, pumpkin seeds, sunflower seeds, chia seeds, flaxseeds; black beans, white beans, kidney beans, chickpeas, pinto beans, lentils (allergies permitting).

Food bowl sauce

Think healthy dressings, or even a ladle of hot, flavourful broth. Chop up some herbs and throw them on top. Is it morning? Go for cinnamon, almond butter, a sprinkling of raw cacao. Next, you'll find some recipes for ugly food bowl sauces.

Ugly food bowl recipes

Remember: preparation is a key part of the Kefir Solution, because the world outside is full of highly processed, high GI, inflammatory foods containing cow's milk, gluten and other baddies. If you go out of the door without taking your food with you, you *will* fall. So here's a week's worth of ugly food bowls to go, or to eat at home.

Variation for vegetarians/vegans: you can swap the meat/fish/egg topping for one of the non-animal protein tryptophan-rich foods listed earlier: fermented soya products, soaked or sprouted legumes (including beans, peas, chickpeas), pumpkin, new or sweet potatoes, cauliflower, mushrooms or leafy greens.

All recipes serve one.

Sunday: salmon and almonds

1 medium salmon fillet

A pinch of dried oregano

Small handful of quinoa and green lentils

1 small avocado, sliced

10 almonds, crushed

1 tbsp sprouted chickpea hummus (*see recipe on page 163*)

Pinch sea salt

Method

1. Preheat the oven to 180°C/350°F/Gas 4.

2. Put the salmon on a sheet of foil, add the oregano and then cook in the oven for 20 minutes.

3. Cover the quinoa and lentils with water, add a pinch of sea salt, bring to the boil and simmer both for 15 minutes.

4. Mix the quinoa and the lentils together, and then place the salmon on top.

5. Add the almonds, avocado and hummus.

6. Serve on a portion of amaranth.

Monday: parma ham and mushrooms

4 slices Parma ham, torn into pieces

7 white cup mushrooms, sliced

2 free-range eggs

8 cubes goat's cheese feta

Handful of spinach and broccoli florets

1 tsp coconut oil

Method

1. Melt the coconut oil in a pan, then add the mushrooms and cook until they start to turn golden.

2. Put the eggs in a pan and start to scramble them. Then throw in the ham, spinach, feta and broccoli, and cook until the feta starts to melt.

3. Layer everything on top of a portion of millet.

Tuesday: tuna and egg

2 eggs

160g/5oz can tuna

1 small avocado, sliced

A few broccoli florets

40g/1½oz goat's cheese feta

Method

1. Soft boil the eggs; throw the broccoli into the water for the last 30 seconds.

2. Layer the eggs/broccoli and the avocado/tuna/feta on top of a portion of millet.

Wednesday: chicken pesto

1 medium chicken fillet

1 sweet potato

1 tbsp green pesto

8 cubes goat's cheese feta

Handful of spinach and broccoli florets

Method

1. Preheat the oven to 200°C/400°F/Gas 6.

2. Cut the sweet potato into fries and bake in the oven for about 35 minutes.

3. Coat the chicken with the pesto and then put it in the oven around 15 minutes after you've added the sweet potato fries.

4. Throw the broccoli and spinach into boiling water for less than a minute.

5. Layer all the ingredients over a portion of buckwheat groats.

Thursday: egg and black turtle beans

Handful of dried black turtle beans

40g/1½oz goat's cheese feta

Handful of spinach

2 hard-boiled eggs

1 tomato, finely chopped

1 tsp coconut oil

A cube of ginger, crushed

½ tsp turmeric

1 tsp coriander

Method

1. The night before, soak the black turtle beans for at least 12 hours; the next day, boil them for 40 minutes.

2. Heat the coconut oil in a pan, then add the ginger, tomato and spices; cook for a few minutes, then pop in the beans and the spinach. Add the feta and eggs.

3. Layer all the ingredients over a portion of amaranth.

Friday: chicken and kidney beans

1 medium chicken breast, cooked

Half 400g can of red kidney beans

Handful of broccoli florets

40g/1½oz goat's cheese feta

Method

1. Boil the kidney beans until they are just lightly cooked through; throw the broccoli florets in with them for the last four minutes.

2. Cut up the chicken and the feta, and add to the beans and broccoli.

3. Layer all the ingredients over a portion of quinoa.

Saturday: chicken, avocado and sweet potato mash

1 medium chicken fillet

1 sweet potato, peeled

1 hard-boiled egg

8 walnuts, crushed

1 small avocado

Paprika

Method

1. Preheat the oven to 200°C/400°F/Gas 6.

2. Cut the sweet potato in half and bake it in the oven alongside the chicken for 30 minutes, or until both are cooked through.

3. Slice the chicken and mash the sweet potato.

4. Cut up the egg and the avocado; mix in the walnuts and then sprinkle paprika over everything.

5. Layer all the ingredients over a portion of millet.

Here are some recipes for the 'sauce' element of your food bowl.

Rocket pesto drizzle

60g/2oz rocket/arugula

30g/1oz shelled pistachios

30g/1oz goat's cheese

2 cloves gut-friendly garlic (*see recipe on page 164*)

½ tsp sea salt

2 tbsp extra virgin olive oil

120ml/4fl oz kefir

Method

1. In a food processor or a high-powered bender, combine the rocket/arugula, pistachios, goat's cheese, garlic and salt. Then drizzle in the olive oil and add the kefir; process until smooth.

2. Scrape out and serve, or store in a tightly covered container for up to a week.

Guacamole

2 ripe avocados

Juice of 1 lime

1 clove gut-friendly garlic (*see recipe on page 164*)

1 tsp sea salt

1 tsp fresh coriander, chopped

Method

1. Use a spoon to scoop the flesh of the avocados into a large bowl. Add the lime juice.

2. With a fork, mash the avocado, garlic and lime until the mixture becomes creamy.

3. Add the sea salt and coriander; mix to combine and serve.

Sprouted chickpea hummus

This raw hummus is prepared so that all of the enzyme inhibitors have been eliminated. This makes it much more nutritious, and easy to digest.

400g/14oz dried chickpeas

1–2 tbsp freshly squeezed lemon juice, to taste (start with less)

2–4 tbsp ground cumin, to taste

2–3 tbsp extra virgin olive oil

4–8 cloves gut-friendly garlic, minced, to taste (*see next recipe*)

1 tsp sea salt, or to taste

1–2 tsp smoked paprika or paprika, to taste

60–120ml/2–4fl oz water

4 tbsp raw tahini or 8 tbsp raw, hulled sesame seeds (optional)

Method

1. Put the chickpeas in a sprouter/jar (*see 'A guide to sprouting' on page 140*), cover them with pure, unchlorinated water and soak for 12 hours.

2. The next day, drain the water from the sprouter/jar and let it sit on the kitchen worktop. Then, twice a day for the next 2-5 days, add water to the chickpeas, swish it around and then drain it out again.

3. Your chickpea sprouts are ready when they have sprouted tiny 'tails' that are around 3mm/⅛ in to 6mm/¼ in long (no longer, or they will taste bad!). Discard any sprouts that turn to mush or rot.

4. Soak the sesame seeds (if using them) for 12 hours prior to making the hummus. Drain and rinse.

5. In a food processor, blend the chickpea sprouts, sesame seeds or tahini (if using), lemon juice, olive oil, garlic, cumin and paprika.

6. Add a little water slowly to the processor, until you start to have a smooth, thick paste. Be slow and conservative, so you don't make the hummus too runny. Add salt to taste, then process until thoroughly smooth and uniform in texture.

7. Garnish with paprika and extra virgin olive oil, and enjoy!

Gut-friendly garlic

Garlic is great stuff, and we all love it – but if you're dealing with IBS, it may not love you. Garlic can be rough on your gut if not properly prepared. But here's a hack for you garlic lovers: you can ferment it to make it gut-friendly. Here's how:

6–8 garlic bulbs (heads)

1 tsp sea salt

1 tbsp kefir

1 tsp dried oregano (optional)

1 bay leaf (optional)

Method

1. Preheat the oven to 100°C/212°F/Gas ¼.

2. Place the whole, unpeeled garlic bulbs on a baking sheet and bake for one hour, or until the cloves begin to pop out of their skins.

3. Leave the bulbs to cool and then remove the cloves from their skins, being careful to leave the ends intact. (Avoid damaging the flesh of the garlic clove, especially on the root end – don't cut it off. Any cuts will cause it to ferment unevenly and make the clove turn blue; that's nothing to worry about: it's just the amino acid reacting with the acid. It won't hurt you, it just looks crazy.)

4. Place the garlic in a 1 litre/1 quart kilner jar with the rest of the ingredients and top with water, leaving 3cm/1 in clear at the top of the jar.

5. Seal loosely and leave on the kitchen worktop for 3–5 days. Then seal tightly and place in the fridge, where it will remain good for six months.

Healthy mayonnaise

2 egg yolks

1 tsp Dijon mustard

1 tbsp lemon juice

50ml/1½fl oz olive oil

200ml/7fl oz vegetable oil

Pinch sea salt and ground black pepper

Method

1. Place the egg yolks, mustard, lemon juice and salt in a small bowl and whisk (using a balloon whisk or electric hand hold whisk) until frothy and combined.

2. Combine the olive oil and vegetable oil in a jug. Pour it very slowly, drop by drop, into the egg mixture, whisking constantly. As the mixture thickens, start adding the oil in a steady stream.

3. Continue until all the oil has been incorporated and the mixture is thick. Season with sea salt and black pepper.

4. Store in an airtight container in the fridge, where it will keep for about seven days.

Other food bowl ideas

You can go conventional with your ugly food bowls. Do you love a tuna-mayo-cheese combo on a baked potato? Try the same topping over quinoa, and run it under the grill – delicious! Or get exotic: try pheasant, goat's cheese and cranberries – why not? As long as it follows the Kefir Solution eating principles, you can mix and match your bowl contents at will.

Cooking your good grains

We're not used to cooking unusual grains in the UK, but it's not a mystery – any grain can be cooked pretty much like rice. Throw it in a pan with water and some salt, and simmer until you like the consistency! If you want to be more scientific about it, here are our recommended cooking times for good grains. Get in the habit of rinsing all grains before cooking, to help remove lectins.

Buckwheat

To cook dried buckwheat groats, rinse them well and then combine with water on the hob in a 2:1 ratio – 475ml/16fl oz water for every 200g/7oz of buckwheat.

Simmer on a low heat for about 20 minutes, checking to see when the groats are plump and their texture is what you're looking for. If they aren't absorbing all the water and appear to become mushy, try straining out some of the water (some people prefer to use 360ml/12fl oz of water to 200g/7oz of buckwheat to prevent this from happening).

200g/7oz buckwheat + 475ml/16fl oz water, cook for 20 minutes – yields 800g/28oz

Millet

To cook millet, you'll need 200g/7oz of raw millet to 625ml/21fl oz of cooking liquid (water or homemade stock). In a large, dry saucepan, toast the raw millet over a medium heat for four to five minutes, or until it turns a rich golden brown and becomes fragrant. Add the water/stock and a pinch of sea salt and stir.

Increase the heat to high and bring the mixture to a boil. Lower the heat and simmer until the grains absorb most of the water; this will take about 15 minutes.

Avoid the temptation to peek a great deal or stir too much (unless the grains stick to the bottom of the pan). Stirring too vigorously will break up the millet and change the texture. Remove the pan from the heat and allow the grains to sit, covered, for 10 minutes. Like most grains, millet needs a little time off the heat to absorb its cooking liquid fully. Fluff with a fork before serving.

200g/7oz millet + 625ml/21fl oz water/stock, cook for 15 minutes, then sit – yields 600g/20oz

Quinoa

To cook quinoa, you'll need 200g/7oz of quinoa to 375ml/12fl oz (water or stock). Bring the quinoa and liquid to a boil in a medium saucepan. Reduce the heat to low, then cover and simmer until tender and most of the liquid has been absorbed; this will take 15 to 20 minutes. Fluff with a fork before serving.

200g/7oz quinoa + 375ml/12fl oz water, cook for 15–20 minutes – yields 500g/16oz

Amaranth

When cooking amaranth grain, use a ratio of 200g/7oz amaranth to 750ml/25fl oz water. Heat the grain/water in a small saucepan until it begins to boil. Then reduce the heat and let it simmer, uncovered, until the water has been absorbed.

200g/7oz amaranth + 750ml/25fl oz water, cook for 25 minutes – yields 600g/20oz

Oats

Any oats are good grains, but the best ones are the least processed! If you have time and patience, go for steel-cut (pinhead) oats. These contain the whole grain, including the oat bran, so are very nutritious.

200g/7oz steel-cut (pinhead) oats + 950ml/32fl oz water, cook for 30 minutes – yields 600g/20oz

If you're tight on time, keep some old-fashioned 'jumbo' rolled oats to hand. These are great for breakfast because they can be cooked very quickly. Use 200g/7oz of oats and 400ml/13fl oz of water, and bring to the boil. Add a pinch of sea salt. Allow to boil, stirring frequently, for five minutes and then remove from the heat. If I have leftover oats from breakfast, I like to smash them into a cake and pan-fry them for a snack later in the day.

Using good grains

Again, the secret here is *preparation*. On a weekend, pick two grains for use as a base for your lunch or supper ugly bowls and cook up a batch. Stash them in the fridge in an airtight container (they will last 3–4 days) and grab alternating scoops for your bowls.

Midweek, cook two different grains in the evening after work... rinse and repeat. Quick and easy! Keep rotating the grains: remember that they all have different nutrients and health benefits, and you want to provide your good bugs with as much variety as possible.

Time-saving hack: cook big batches of your favourite grains and allow them to cool completely. Freeze in appropriately sized portions in zip-top freezer bags. You can defrost the grains in the fridge overnight, or on the kitchen worktop for a few hours, before reheating.

On the farm, we're not big fans of microwaves, so I reheat everything in a saucepan. But do what works for you! Steaming the grains works well to reheat them, or you can pan sauté them in a bit of goat's butter or olive oil – extra delicious.

Supper

Here's a week's of worth of inspiration for meals that follow the Kefir Solution eating principles. Each recipe serves four.

Sunday: roast chicken

I love to roast a free-range chicken on a Sunday: it's a beautiful, healthy, traditional meal that's rich in tryptophan and a real crowd-pleaser. A free-range bird is more expensive than a regular one, but you can justify the additional cost by making a chicken soup on Monday – that way, you're getting two meals out of it!

1 free-range chicken

16–20 new potatoes, peeled

4 carrots, peeled and roughly chopped

2 parsnips, peeled and roughly chopped

Extra virgin olive oil

Sea salt and pepper

Optional fresh herbs – rosemary, sage, bay

Method

1. Preheat the oven to 200°C/400°F/Gas 6.

2. If you have fresh herbs around, make a bouquet with them, tied with twine, and insert it into the chicken's cavity. Rosemary, sage and bay are nice.

3. Put the chicken in a roasting tin, and sprinkle its skin with olive oil, sea salt and pepper. Pour 250ml/8fl oz of water into the roasting pan. Cover the chicken with foil.

4. Surround the chicken with the new potatoes and rough-cut carrots and parsnips. Sprinkle with olive oil, and season with sea salt and pepper.

5. Put the roasting tin in the oven and cook the chicken and potatoes for 1–2 hours, depending on the weight of the chicken. For the last 30 minutes of cooking, remove the foil so the bird's skin can crisp.

Save the carcass, the bones and all the leftover bits, including any vegetables – you'll be using it all tomorrow to make chicken soup!

Monday: chicken soup

This is the ultimate Kefir Solution food. It's rich in tryptophan and has loads of healthy veg; simmering the chicken bones adds lots of lovely gut-healing collagen, too. For this recipe, you'll need the roast chicken carcass from Sunday.

1 free-range chicken carcass (with leftover meat attached)

8 carrots

16 new potatoes

1 onion

1 swede

1 leek

2 tsp sea salt

5 whole black peppercorns

Method

1. Put the chicken carcass into a big saucepan. Add water until it's about 5cm/2 in from the top of the pan. Bring the water

to the boil, then lower the heat and simmer the carcass for at least two hours. The longer the better!

2. Sieve out the bones and the meat from the broth. I do this by tipping the whole lot into a second large pan, with a colander sitting in it. The meat and bones go into the colander, while the broth percolates through to the second pan.

3. Put the broth back onto the heat, and continue simmering. Add all the vegetables to the broth. I use those listed previously, but you can try whatever your family likes. They can all be chopped quite roughly, in big pieces – this is a hearty peasant-style soup. Simmer the vegetables in the broth for about an hour.

4. Place the meat and bones in the colander to one side, to allow the whole thing to cool down. Once the meat and bones have cooled enough to handle comfortably, pick any remaining meat off the carcass. It should now come away easily. Add the meat back into the pot 15 minutes before serving.

5. To give the soup a traditional Welsh feel, chop a leek and toss it in 15 minutes before you're ready to serve. Season to taste with more sea salt and black pepper.

Tuesday: pork delish in a dish

After two days of chicken, you and your gut bugs will be ready for another kind of meat. Why eat pork? The National Geographic Blue Zones study noted that pork is one of the foods common to all of the Blue Zones, which are regions and countries boasting the most centenarians.[5] Plus, as we know, it's rich in tryptophan, which is going to make your gut and your brain happy!

4 bone-in pork chops

2 sweet potatoes

1 fennel bulb

1 bunch asparagus

2 firm peaches or apples

2 tsp chopped sage, rosemary or thyme

4 tbsp apple cider vinegar

150ml/5fl oz chicken stock (homemade or from a stock cube)

Sea salt and freshly ground black pepper

2 tsp Dijon mustard

4 tbsp coconut oil

Method

1. Preheat the oven to 175°C/350°F/Gas 4.

2. Peel the sweet potatoes, cut them in half lengthwise and slice into ½-cm/¼-inch rounds.

3. Slice the fennel lengthwise into eight wedges, including stems and fronds.

4. Cut the peaches or apples into eight pieces.

5. Snap the ends off the asparagus and halve the spears.

6. Season the pork chops and sweet potato with salt and pepper.

7. Heat the coconut oil in a large ovenproof pan over a medium–high heat. Brown the chops and sweet potato, turning once (about three minutes each side).

8. Remove the chops from the pan briefly, and add the fennel, asparagus, peach or apple, and the herbs. Stir to combine,

then return the chops to the pan, putting them on top of the veggies, fruit and herbs.

9. Combine the cider vinegar, stock and mustard together in a jug, and then pour over everything in the pan. Put a lid on the pan and cook in the oven for 15 minutes.

Wednesday: Gemma's Mediterranean turkey with lemon kefir sauce

This recipe is from one of our beloved Chuckling Goat clients: thanks, Gemma! It's a simple yet yummy dish that's perfect for when you don't have lots of time but want a very nourishing meal. Turkey is a tryptophan high-performer, and we don't eat enough of it – it's not just for Christmas anymore.

680g/1lb 5oz organic minced (ground) dark turkey (thigh meat). It's also delicious with 450g/1lb organic grass-fed minced (ground) beef or buffalo, or grass-fed lamb

2–3 cloves gut-friendly garlic, minced (*see recipe on page 164*)

Half an organic onion

1 tbsp organic, unfiltered, raw apple cider vinegar

120ml/4fl oz bone broth (chicken or beef); preferably homemade, but a cube is fine

Courgette/zucchini, carrot and celery stalk: one of each

Pitted black and green olives: five of each

120ml/4fl oz kefir

Juice of half an organic lemon or 1 tsp lemon zest

1 tbsp extra virgin olive oil

1–2 tbsp avocado oil

Salt and pepper to taste

Method

1. Dice the courgette/zucchini, carrot, celery stalk and onion.

2. In a pan, sauté the minced garlic and onion in the avocado oil. Once browned, add the meat and sauté until just cooked through.

3. Add the apple cider vinegar, bone broth, vegetables and olives to the pan. Simmer for 5–10 minutes.

4. Turn off the heat and mix in the olive oil. Add salt and pepper to taste.

5. Mix the kefir with the lemon juice/zest and drizzle over the meat after serving.

This is great served in a big bowl over a bed of mixed organic greens, organic Japanese or purple sweet potato, half an organic avocado and a big scoop of organic sauerkraut.

Thursday: beef stew

This is a warming, tender beef stew packed with lovely chunky root veg. I'm a big fan of slow cooking – put this in the slow cooker in the morning before you leave for work, and it will be waiting for you, perfuming the air with gorgeous scents, when you come home!

800g/1lb 7oz stewing steak or beef skirt

2 parsnips

1 onion

500g/1lb 2oz new potatoes

Half a butternut squash

Handful of Jerusalem artichokes

4 carrots

1 lemon

A few sprigs of fresh sage and rosemary

Plain flour

2 tbsp tomato purée

1 clove of gut-friendly garlic (*see recipe on page 164*)

Half a bottle of red wine

Olive oil and knob of unsalted butter, for frying

285ml/10fl oz organic beef or vegetable stock

Method

1. Preheat the oven to 160°C/300°F/Gas 2.

2. Cut the beef into 5cm/2 in pieces

3. Peel and roughly chop the onion, peel and quarter the parsnips and peel and halve the carrots. Deseed and roughly dice the squash, and peel and halve the Jerusalem artichokes. Pick the sage leaves.

4. Heat a little olive oil and the butter in a casserole pan on a medium heat. Add the onion and the sage leaves and fry for 3–4 minutes.

5. Meanwhile, toss the beef in a little seasoned flour, then add it to the pan with all the vegetables, the tomato purée, the wine and stock, and gently stir together. Season generously with black pepper and just a little sea salt.

6. Bring to the boil, then put a lid on the pan and place it in the oven. Cook until the meat is tender; sometimes this takes

three hours, sometimes four – it depends on which cut of meat you're using and how fresh it is. The only way to test it is to mash up a piece of meat and if it falls apart easily, it's ready.

7. Once the stew is cooked, turn the oven down to 110°C/225°F/ Gas ¼ and just hold the pan there until you're ready to eat.

8. Zest the lemon, pick and finely chop the rosemary and finely chop the garlic, then mix together and sprinkle over the stew before serving.

The best way to serve this is by ladling big spoonfuls of it into bowls and accompanying it with some really fresh, warmed kefir soda bread (*see recipe on page 153*).

Friday: crunchy almond chicken

We're back to chicken today, because let's face it: most of us love chicken! It's rich in tryptophan, and not as heavy on the system as red meat. Got to keep the variety rotation going, to feed those gut bugs.

6 chicken thighs or drumsticks

285g/10oz sugar snap peas

A bunch of asparagus

100g/3½oz natural almond butter

1 tbsp coconut oil, melted

2 tbsp tamari

1 tsp dried chilli flakes

1 clove gut-friendly garlic (*see recipe on page 164)*

2-cm/¾-in knob of ginger

2 tbsp fresh rosemary

4 tbsp flaked almonds

1 lime

2 tbsp white sesame seeds, sprouted

Method

1. Preheat the oven to 170°C/325°F/Gas 3.

2. Mince the garlic clove and the ginger. Snap the ends of the asparagus and halve the spears; cut the lime into wedges.

3. In a baking tray, combine the almond butter, coconut oil, tamari, chilli, garlic and ginger, and mix well.

4. Add the chicken and toss around to coat. Place in the oven and bake for 15 minutes.

5. Remove the chicken from the oven and arrange the vegetables, rosemary, almonds, lime wedges and sesame seeds around and over the chicken.

6. Return the tray to the oven and cook for another 15 minutes, or until the chicken is fully browned and crispy.

Serve with the following side dish featuring Jerusalem artichoke (hello, resistant starch!)

Crispy roasted Jerusalem artichokes

800g/1lb 7oz Jerusalem artichokes

1 garlic bulb (head)

1 tbsp rosemary leaves, chopped

3 tbsp olive oil

Pinch ground mace

30g/1oz butter

2 tsp lemon juice

Method

1. Preheat the oven to 180°C/350°F/Gas 4.

2. Cut the garlic bulb in half, down the middle.

3. Soak the artichokes in cold water for 20 minutes or so to loosen any dirt, then scrub them with a scourer, being sure to remove any grit. Halve the small ones and quarter the bigger ones, and then put them in a roasting tin with the split garlic bulb and rosemary. Coat everything with the olive oil and season.

4. Roast for 45–50 minutes until the veg/garlic are tender inside and crispy outside.

5. To finish, squeeze the softened garlic cloves from their skins and toss with the roasted artichokes, along with the mace, butter and lemon juice.

Saturday: quinoa fishcakes

500g/1lb new potatoes

100g/3½oz quinoa

3 × 200g/7oz smoked mackerel fillets, skin removed

1 bunch of fresh parsley

Half a bunch of fresh tarragon

1 large free-range egg

⅔ tsp chilli flakes

2½ lemons

Olive oil

Method

1. Preheat the oven to 190°C/375°F/Gas 5.

2. Simmer the new potatoes in salted water for 20 minutes, until cooked through. Roughly mash, with the skins. Set aside to cool.

3. Put the quinoa in a small pan, cover it with 185ml/6fl oz water and bring to the boil; simmer for 15 minutes or so until it's cooked but still al dente. Drain the quinoa and then stir it through the potato.

4. Put 3 tbsp of olive oil in a frying pan and place over a medium–high heat. Add the chilli flakes and stir for one minute before adding to the potato/quinoa mixture.

5. With a fork, flake the mackerel into small pieces. Pick the leaves from the herbs and roughly chop them; beat the egg.

6. Add the fish, herbs and egg to the potato/quinoa mixture, along with the zest of 1½ lemons, ¾ tsp salt and a few twists of ground black pepper.

7. Mix to combine, then shape into 12 cakes, around 3cm/1 in thick, and set aside.

8. Heat 2 tbsp olive oil in a large frying pan. When hot, add six of the fishcakes and fry for 3–4 minutes, or until golden on both sides, turning halfway through.

9. Remove the fishcakes from the pan and place them on a lined baking tray. Add another tablespoon of oil to the pan and cook the remaining six cakes.

10. Put the fishcakes in the oven for around eight minutes, or
    until cooked through. Cut the remaining lemons into wedges
    and serve with the fishcakes.

This is delicious served with a big green salad studded with beetroot
and carrot.

The Super Supper Smoothie

Now, I have two non-vegetable loving guys in the house, and
although they're quite happy to chow down on meat and root
veggies like carrots, swede and new potatoes, it's often quite
difficult to entice them to eat dark leafy greens. No problem – my
Super Supper Smoothie comes to the rescue! Easier, quicker and
less of an argument than a side helping of greens, it goes on the
supper table in a little juice glass.

We have two daily smoothies on the farm – the overnight kefir
oats one (*see breakfast section on page 146*) and the Super Supper
Smoothie to eat alongside the evening meal. The suppertime
smoothie is my insurance policy really: it allows me to sneak
the extra dark leafy greens into the boys' diet that they might
otherwise leave on the plate.

I can also shovel in some fruit, toss in some inulin-containing
Jerusalem artichoke and even add the odd beetroot – they never
know the difference. And the beauty of the Super Supper Smoothie
is that once you blend those leafy greens up with fruit, it looks
green, but tastes pink! They will slurp down those veggies with
nary a whimper. This is one of the many reasons why I suggest you
treat yourself to a high-powered blender. Anything that's difficult
to eat, simply stick it in a smoothie, whizz it up and you're done.

Super Supper Smoothie ideas

Here's a week's worth of suggestions for your supper smoothies; the quantities serve one

Monday

A handful of chard; 2 stalks of celery; half a banana; 100g/3½oz papaya

Tuesday

A handful of spinach; 100g/3½oz shredded cabbage; 100g/3½oz pineapple; half an avocado

Wednesday

A handful of lettuce; 1 small apple, cored; 1 kiwi; 1 carrot

Thursday

A handful of carrot tops; 1 carrot; 1 beetroot (raw or cooked); 100g/3½oz blueberries; 1 orange, peeled

Friday

A handful of rocket/arugula; 15g/½oz peeled ginger root; a small handful of fresh oregano; 100g/3½oz watermelon; 1 ripe pear

Saturday

A handful of beet tops; half a beetroot; 1 orange, peeled; 1 small apple, cored; 100g/3½oz Jerusalem artichoke

Sunday

100g/3½oz romaine lettuce; 100g/3½oz shredded cabbage; 1 banana; 100g/3½oz blueberries; half an avocado

Rotate your greens

Keeping in mind the concept of biodiversity in the microbiome, it's important that you rotate the dark leafy greens in your Super Supper Smoothie, so you have a variety of veg making its way down into your gut ecosystem.

Basically, all plants contain small amounts of toxins to ensure their longevity: that way, when animals graze on them, they're encouraged to move on to a different pasture and type of plant before one type becomes extinct. In small amounts, these toxins aren't harmful to humans, but if we consume enough of them, they can cause problems. For example, the oxalates in spinach can cause kidney stones.

Typically, you wouldn't eat enough of any leafy green veg to really run into a problem. But with green smoothies, you're packing a ton of greens into each serving because the blender massively compresses them. If you're consuming several portions of greens daily, you'll want to rotate them to ensure you're achieving the maximum amount of health benefits – and the least amount of toxins.

There are four families of leafy green vegetables, and the plants in each family are genetically quite similar to each other. So to get the best effect, rotate between families. The first type, *Brassicaceae*, includes kale, spring cabbage, rocket/arugula, bok choy and mustard greens.

The second family, *Amaranthaceae*, includes spinach, chard and beet; the third, *Asteraceae*, includes dandelion leaves, lettuce and chicory; and the fourth, *Apiaceae*, includes carrot tops and parsley.

How often do you need to rotate the greens in your Super Supper Smoothies? There's no need to be strict about it: once a week or so is fine. The goal is to avoid buying the same greens – spinach, say – for weeks, or even months, on end. In the real world, you may choose to buy one type of leafy green per week, and then rotate to a new one the following week, which is fine. The ideas included previously are just a concept example, to get you into the idea of rotating your greens.

Trying to lose weight? Just have the Super Supper Smoothie and skip the meat and root vegetable bit of supper. You'll still be getting great nutrition, and you'll be surprised how quickly the weight comes off.

As I said earlier, the great thing about smoothies as opposed to juicing is that they contain all the fibre of the fruit or vegetable. This slows down the rate at which the food is burned inside your system, lowering its GI impact. So when you're consuming a fruit or veg, always eat it whole or blended – never juiced, with all that helpful pulp taken out!

Treats

So, while you're following the Kefir Solution, which food and drink can you have as a treat? First off, let the trumpets sound – chocolate! But keep in mind that this is *real* chocolate, not milk chocolate. I'm talking about raw cacao, or chocolate that has 70 per cent or greater cocoa solids, which is known to contain tryptophan.[6]

You can have one square of this in the evening – you'll find that it's not 'moreish' in the way that milk chocolate is, because it doesn't have all the bad stuff that gets you right in the dopamine cycle. The best thing for you really is raw cacao nibs or powder.

Just to be super clear on this one: real chocolate contains both serotonin and tryptophan. Milk chocolate, on the other hand, contains a lower amount of cocoa solids, and therefore a lower concentration of the psychoactive compounds that we're after to make us happy. Milk chocolate is also full of sugar – which creates dopamine – and that's going to decrease your precious tryptophan.[7]

So, 70 per cent chocolate or raw cacao powder = good. Milk chocolate = bad.

Here's some more good news: in recent studies, wine, coffee and tea were all found to boost the biodiversity in our microbiome. So you can indulge in these treats – sensibly, of course![8] Don't sweeten your coffee or tea with sugar: 100 per cent pure stevia is best for that. If you like to add milk, use goat's milk or another acceptable non-cow alternative: oat, almond and rice milks are all okay, but not soy.

Opt for red wine, as it has health-boosting resveratrol, and keep your intake moderate – ideally one small glass per day. Dr Claudia Kawas and her team at the University of California investigated why some people reach 90 years of age and beyond, and others don't. Their study showed that the daily habits of people who lived past 90 included drinking coffee, getting out of the house, talking to neighbours, having a positive attitude, getting 15 minutes of exercise and drinking a glass of wine to destress.[9]

Interestingly, many of these habits are serotonin boosters, and they definitely make life more fun: so enjoy them!

With that in mind, here's a little something designed to fight those late afternoon energy dips. Invite a friend over for coffee and share the goodies!

Shann's SuperPower Mocha

1 tsp raw cacao powder

1 tsp Siberian ginseng powder

1 tsp gotu kola powder

Method

1. Mix the powders into a paste with a little hot water. Top with one large mug of coffee of your choice, adding goat's milk if you wish. I use my latte maker to steam up a goat's milk latte.

2. Stir to incorporate the goodies at the bottom of the mug, then top with a dusting of cinnamon. And zing – away you go!

Note: the taste of this drink is bitter – from the both the coffee and the raw cacao powder – as I haven't added any sweetener to the recipe. Bitter is good. Bitter improves your digestion. Learn to embrace bitter!

Here's a little information about two of the ingredients in the SuperPower Mocha:

Siberian ginseng

Eleutherococcius senticosus, commonly known as Siberian ginseng, is something of a wonder plant. In the 1960s the Soviet government did extensive research on it, developing it in order to boost the immune system of its workers in Siberia.

A huge amount of science has been done since on this potent adaptogen, including its ability to improve digestion, increase strength, relieve lethargy and bloating from weak digestion and improve memory and concentration; it also has a powerful anti-fatigue effect that increases endurance and the ability of the mitochondria in our cells to produce energy.

Gotu kola

Hydrocotyle asiatica, or gotu kola, is a well-known brain tonic that's used to treat depletion by stress and anxiety, insomnia and depression; it also calms mental turbulence. It's good for indigestion, acidity and ulcers, too.[10]

Siberian ginseng and gotu kola are both nourishing remedies: take one teaspoon of each daily, in goat's milk (or kefir), to help replenish the system.

Avoid gotu kola during pregnancy and while breastfeeding. I personally prefer to take the powdered root of gotu kola, instead of an extract of it in a capsule, as the root powder is closer to the actual form of the plant, and is harder to overconsume.

Speak with your GP if you're currently taking other medications, as these herbs may interfere with prescription drugs.

Chapter 12

The Kefir Solution Step #5:
Make Lifestyle Shifts

Now we have the main elements of the programme in place, and you are:

- Drinking kefir

- Taking ashwagandha

- Leaning in to your feelings

- Adopting new eating habits

So, what further lifestyle changes can you make, to really drive the beneficial effects of this programme forward?

Drink medical herbal tea

Medical herbs are a powerful, natural way to treat symptoms of IBS, depression and anxiety. We've created an awful lot of problems with our overuse of chemicals and toxins, but generously, Nature offers us a solution to those – with 'medical' herbs. Herbs are fabulous. Herbs are wonderful. I love herbs. And here's why:

A medical herb will have a multiplicity of good effects on your system. Take meadowsweet, as just one example. Meadowsweet contains salicylic acid, which is the active painkiller ingredient in aspirin. We humans think we're so clever: lookee, we've isolated the active component of the plant, put it in a pill and put it up for sale!

But... isolating that compound has created a bit of a nightmare. Aspirin will ease your headache and thin your blood, but it may also have harmful side-effects: it inhibits helpful substances that protect the stomach's delicate lining, creating the risk of stomach upset or bleeding in the stomach and intestines. Not ideal.

The herb meadowsweet, on the other hand, not only gives you the painkilling punch of salicylic acid, but is also antacid, antibacterial, prevents vomiting, is anti-inflammatory, antispasmodic, astringent, a diuretic, a relaxant, promotes appetite, assists digestion and acts as a urinary antiseptic.

Meadowsweet has numerous beneficial effects for systems in your body, including your digestion, your skin, your mental and emotional state, your musculoskeletal system, your immune system and your skin. So, which form of painkiller would *you* rather take?

Each medical herb has numerous benefits for many of your body systems. Why so many, and so good? Because plants have been at this bacteria-fighting exercise for 15 billion years, and they've become really good at it.

Plants can't run away, so they've had to develop multiple levels of defence against any virus or bug that happens along. And we humans have evolved alongside plants: our immune systems are designed to coordinate with theirs, and vice versa.

All those components that we strip out in the chemical process of creating a pharmaceutical are there in the plant for a reason. Why get rid of them, when they can help us?

Shann's medical teas

Here's a selection of my own medical herbal tea recipes, developed over time to help my family, clients and team members. I encourage you to explore the wonderful world of medical herbs for yourself. Each plant serves a wide variety of helpful functions, and will give you powerful tools to enhance your own and your family's health!

I order all my herbs from a reputable supplier (*see Resources section*) and store them in a dry, dark place. This is the method I use to make all my teas:

1. Combine one teaspoon of each herb in a teapot or saucepan, cover with 720ml/24fl oz of freshly boiled water, replace the lid, and steep for 15 minutes.

2. Strain and drink one cup, three times a day.

I've listed the functions of each herb in the following recipes, to help give you a sense of how the plants work in combination with one another.[1]

Dry it up tea

Helpful for diarrhoea

- **Yarrow** – dries up secretions and tones the gut

- **Agrimony** – an astringent digestive tonic

- **Marshmallow root** – soothes irritation

- **Chamomile** – reduces anxiety in stress-related diarrhea; also an anti-spasmodic

Get it going tea

Helpful for constipation. (Here we see the original reason for the creation of 'Dandelion and Burdock' drinks!)

- **Dandelion root** – a mild laxative

- **Burdock root** – its mucilaginous fibres absorb toxins and enhance bowel elimination

- **Yellow dock root** – stimulates peristalsis and cleanses the bowel

Sing me to sleep tea

Drink this 30 minutes before bedtime

- **Valerian** – a relaxant

- **Lavender** – combats bowel problems related to anxiety

- **Hops** – a mild sedative

- **Chamomile** – an anti-spasmodic

Settle my tummy tea

- **Meadowsweet** – this offers mild pain relief

- **Peppermint** – an anti-inflammatory

- **Rosemary** – relieves wind and bloating

- **Marshmallow root** – soothes irritation

Get me through the day tea

- **Rosemary** – calms anxiety and lifts depression

- **Mugwort** – a stimulant and tonic; also helps prevent infection

- **Vervain** – soothes irritation and supports the body during stress

- **Peppermint** – a brain tonic

Calm me down tea

- **Rose petals** – uplifting and calming

- **Lavender** – helps relieve agitation

- **Calendula** – reduces inflammation

- **Chamomile** – calms anxiety and tension

Take collagen

One of the most important things you can do to heal your IBS, depression and anxiety, after adding kefir to your diet, is to take a daily collagen supplement.

Collagen is quite literally the 'glue' that holds our bodies together. It's the most abundant protein in our bodies – it's found in the tendons, bones, muscles, skin, blood vessels and most importantly for IBS sufferers, in the digestive system.

We're born with lots of collagen. Think of the lovely plump, peachy skin a baby has – that's collagen at its finest! Sadly, our collagen production begins to slow down around the age of 30, right around the time those first lines and wrinkles start to appear.

After the age of 30, our collagen level drops by 1–2 per cent every year. By the age of 40, we've lost 10–20 per cent of our collagen. By the age of 50, we're down 20–40 per cent. And by 60? Well, you can imagine... and it's not pretty!

Collagen and the gut

After the age of 50, our epithelium starts to develop holes and tears that the body struggles to mend, *because it lacks collagen*. More than 50 per cent of the population aged over 60 develops something called 'pouches' in the lining of the colon. Occasionally these pouches can become inflamed, leading to diverticulitis, which causes pain and infection in the abdomen. Doctors usually treat it with antibiotics, or, in more severe cases, surgery.

After a bout of diverticulitis, many folks feel like a different person – and not in a good way. They report ongoing IBS symptoms such as recurrent abdominal pain, cramping and diarrhoea that they didn't have before. Most doctors tend to wave this off, insisting that once the diverticulitis is gone, it's gone. Now, finally, research has acknowledged that diverticulitis can be an inflammatory process – like a bomb going off in the body and leaving residual damage.

Scientists undertaking one study reported a major surprise: diverticulitis patients not only developed IBS at a higher rate than the controls, but they also developed mood disorders like depression and anxiety at a higher rate. Because IBS and mood disorders go hand in hand, this suggests that acute diverticulitis might set off a process leading to long-standing changes in the gut–brain axis.[2] You can just imagine the havoc that wreaks inside your system!

Where to find collagen

So, you've got to consume collagen. And when I say consume, I mean take it every day, religiously. You've absolutely got to have it in your system, so your body can repair the holes and tears in your gut.

Collagen and kefir work together in a marvellous one-two healing tango – collagen heals the lining of the gut, and the kefir repopulates it with the good bugs it needs to get your serotonin system singing again.

Inside the gut, collagen helps forms connective tissue – sealing and healing the protective lining of the GI tract. Studies have found that in patients with inflammatory bowel disease, serum concentrations of collagen are decreased.[3] Collagen also helps with the absorption of water within the intestines, keeping things moving more freely out of body.

Collagen is super important, and you need to consume it! So how are we going to get it into your body? For a while I was advocating bone broth. Collagen lurks in a lot of foods that our ancestors used to eat and cook with, but which today we mostly throw away – bones, tendons and gristly bits.

Bones are loaded with collagen, and as the bones simmer in broth during the cooking process that takes place over one to two days, the collagen slowly breaks down into gelatin – the cooked form of collagen. If you then consume the bone broth, you ingest all that collagen goodness.

So, bone broth is terrific! However, after some real-world analysis, I found that our clients just weren't carrying through with the bone broth every day. Too much hassle. I get it! We're all busy.

But it's *so* important that you have collagen every single day, that I now recommend taking a high-quality collagen supplement. You can find it in a powder that can be mixed into hot or cold drinks. It's relatively odourless and tasteless, so it's simple enough to take it consistently, day in, day out.

Personally, I take my collagen powder by adding one tablespoon of it to a mug, adding hot water, then finishing with a pinch of sea salt and a squeeze of lemon.

Apart from helping with IBS, depression and anxiety – as it repairs your gut lining – you'll notice other nifty benefits to taking a daily collagen supplement: firmer, smoother skin, a reduction in cellulite and stretchmarks, less joint pain, increased metabolism, improved energy levels, better wound healing, stronger nails, teeth and hair, better liver and artery health, and improved circulation.[4] What's not to love?

Take vitamin D and omega-3 fatty acids

Research shows that dietary intervention with vitamin D, tryptophan and omega-3 fatty acids boosts brain serotonin concentrations.[5] Why is that? It's because we need vitamin D and omega-3 fatty acids to *allow* the tryptophan to be converted into serotonin.[6]

Doing so is a challenge, though, because official estimates suggest that in England, one in five adults and one in six children may have low levels of both vitamin D and omega-3.

Vitamin D

Widespread vitamin D deficiency is a big part of the IBS problem. Recent British research shows that up to 82 per cent of IBS sufferers have insufficient levels of vitamin D, and data suggests that supplementing the vitamin can reduce symptoms.[7]

Ideally, we'd all get enough vitamin D from the action of sunlight on our skin, but this isn't always possible; in 2016, government health officials advised that the British population should consume 10mg of vitamin D daily in the autumn and winter, when sunshine is scarce.[8] The Mayo Clinic in the USA recommends 10mg of vitamin D for children up to age 12 months, 15mg for ages 1 to 70 years, and 20mg for those aged 70 and over.

You're going to get much of this through drinking kefir – 100ml/3fl oz of kefir contains 2.5mg of vitamin D, so the recommended daily dose of 170ml/6fl oz of kefir will give you nearly half of your daily allowance. You should consider taking an additional vitamin D supplement for the remaining 5mg of vitamin D that you need.

Omega-3 fatty acids

This is super important, and it's possible you're not getting enough of it. Omega-3 is commonly discussed in conjunction with oily fish, but here's the kicker if you're hoping to use oily fish as a source: the omega-3 comes from algae, not the fish itself.

If the fish eats the algae, the fish will contain the omega-3. But only *wild* fish eat algae. Farmed fish don't eat algae – they eat pellets. This is why you'll often see the recommendation to eat 'wild-caught' fish.

To be honest, this is just way too much of a headache for me. I'm all for simplicity, so I go straight for an omega-3 algae oil. These are oils that were developed when researchers finally understood that the right kind of omega-3 came from the algae, and not from the fish: so why not just head for the source?

Make sure that the algae oil supplement you choose has more EPA than DHA (two different types of long-chain fatty acids). The label should display this information. How much omega-3 should we take? Studies have shown that high doses, from 200–2,200mg per day, can reduce symptoms of depression and anxiety.[9] And now you understand why! Do not exceed 3,000mg of omega-3 per day.

Which other supplements are useful?

I prefer to get everything I need from my diet and natural sources, like kefir, root powders or herbal teas. But you may find that your Kefir Solution results stall, or that you need an extra push to deal with an acute condition related to your IBS. In that case, I recommend the following natural supplements to give you a boost.

L-glutamine

L-glutamine is the major fuel source for cells in the small intestine. This amino acid supports gut function and improves gastrointestinal health because it's a vital nutrient for the intestines to rebuild and repair.[10] L-glutamine improves IBS and diarrhoea by balancing mucus production, which results in healthy bowel movements.[11]

It's important to know that the majority of people don't get enough L-glutamine from their food alone, so supplementation is a good idea. Typically, the best daily dose is between 500 and 1500mg.

Iron

Iron is required to synthesize both serotonin and dopamine, and serotonin receptors are known to regulate iron-carrying proteins.[12] Milk kefir contains lactoferrin, a substance that helps your body to absorb and process iron, so an iron supplement in combination with your kefir is going to get the job done properly. I like to take a liquid iron supplement that also contains an array of B vitamins, like Feroglobin; these are gentle on the system.

Avoid antacids and PPIs

If you have indigestion after eating a meal, it may feel as if you have too much stomach acid. So you reach for an antacid to reduce the amount of acid. Acid indigestion, right?

Wrong. Antacids and PPIs (proton pump inhibitors) like Omeprazole can work against you, and here's why: generally, the biggest factor in indigestion is not too much stomach acid, but too *little*.

The importance of stomach acid

Here's a very quick rundown of how digestion works: while chewing your food begins the mechanical and chemical breakdown process of digestion, the real heavy lifting is done by the stomach. Specifically, protein triggers the release of stomach acid (hydrochloric acid, or HCl). HCl is a very strong acid designed to 'get things going' and break everything down to a point where it can pass along to the small intestine.

Food isn't supposed to remain in the stomach for very long: the HCl should be strong enough to break it down, and move it along to the duodenum. When the HCl isn't strong enough, or there isn't enough of it to go around, food stays in the stomach for longer than it should. Proteins putrefy, carbohydrates start to ferment, and you experience bloating, discomfort and gas that 'refluxes' back into the oesophagus.

Another reason that you need strong stomach acid is this: your body has a natural feedback loop that's trying to protect you from nasty pathogens that cause infection inside your gut. You're absorbing these bad guys all the time, in your food and water.

When bad bacteria get into your system, it responds with inflammation, which is a protective response. This triggers the production of more HCl, which kills off the invading microbes. Shut down your gastric acid production, and you're messing with your stomach's natural defence mechanism, leaving it vulnerable and without protection. And what can result from this? Chronic gastritis, which if left untreated can lead to peptic ulcers and stomach cancer.[13]

Look at it from your digestive system's point of view: your poor body is desperately trying to *protect* you from your own risky behaviour, as you're consuming all sorts of bad bacteria, all the time. So there's a defensive HCl wash in your stomach, carefully designed to be strong enough to kill those baddies off and keep you safe. And then you go popping pills that deactivate the strength of that protective acid wash. Well, it's enough to drive a stomach to tears. Literally!

If you're popping antacids and PPIs to weaken the strength of that protective acid bath, then you can't blame your stomach when the invaders just waltz straight in and take over. You've killed off your own defenders, and handed over the keys to the city to the gastrointestinal Vikings.

After conducting two new studies on mice, scientists at the University of Michigan Medical School in the USA found that 'reduced gastric acidity does appear to make the mammalian stomach more vulnerable to bacterial invasion and gastritis. Juanita L. Merchant, one of the study authors, says that 'physicians may want to re-evaluate the long-term use of omeprazole and other proton pump-inhibiting drugs in their patients.'[14]

So acid-reducing and blocking drugs are just sticking plasters that do nothing to address the underlying cause of the problem. In fact, they may make things worse: by suppressing the symptoms and allowing you to carry on eating as you were, they may lay the foundations for some serious long-term health complications.

Low stomach acid and IBS

In the whole IBS-depression-anxiety scenario, this is particularly harmful. Remember that tryptophan that you need to make serotonin? Well, if your stomach acid isn't strong enough, you can't break proteins down properly, and you won't be able to absorb tryptophan. So there's a logical link between low stomach acid and depression, anxiety and other debilitating mood imbalances.

And that's not all. Before reaching for that daily antacid or PPI, spare a thought for what it's doing to your poor gut bugs! In the USA, a Mayo Clinic study showed that people who regularly take PPIs have less diversity among their gut bacteria, putting them at increased risk for infections like *Clostridium difficile* and pneumonia, in addition to vitamin deficiencies and bone fractures.[15]

John DiBaise, a Mayo Clinic gastroenterologist and a senior author on the study, says: 'Evidence has been mounting for years that long-term use of inhibitors poses increased risks for a variety of associated complications, but we have never really understood why. What this study does for the first time is demonstrate a plausible explanation for these associated conditions.'[16]

Dr DiBaise says that 'diet, genetics and environmental exposure all play a role in maintaining a healthy microbiome, which is critical to overall wellness. Significant changes to the microbiome, like those caused by proton pump inhibitors, can put people at risk for over-colonization by undesirable species.'[17]

Many epidemiological studies have linked PPIs to nutritional, metabolic and infectious disorders, despite the drugs' long history of safety and efficacy. Specifically, their prolonged use has been associated with iron and vitamin B12 deficiencies, hypomagnesemia, osteoporosis-related fractures, small intestinal bacterial overgrowth, and community-acquired pneumonia.

The US Food and Drug Administration has issued several safety communications about use of high-dose PPIs (available through prescription) and long-term use at any dose, including over-the-counter medications.[18]

Alternative therapies for acid indigestion

So what can you do instead? Try these three natural remedies:

Apple cider vinegar + bitters before meals

Take one tablespoon of apple cider vinegar 'with the mother' in a small amount of water immediately before meals. Apple cider vinegar with the mother is simply unrefined, unpasteurized and unfiltered apple cider vinegar. The 'mother' is a colony of beneficial bacteria, similar to kefir grains, that helps create vinegar through a secondary fermentation process. This is a great natural remedy because apple cider vinegar has a very low pH in balance with your stomach.

You can also add one teaspoon of bitters to this mix. Bitters comes in a tincture, and they do what it says on the tin: they taste bitter! This bitter taste stimulates your liver and gall bladder to produce high-quality bile, which will help you digest your food.

As a flavour, 'bitter' has fallen out of favour in today's palate. Of the five major flavours – sweet, bitter, sour, salty, umami (or savoury) – bitter rarely gets a look-in. We're big on sweet and salty, but even the vegetables in the supermarket have been bred to eliminate bitterness! This is a pity, as studies have shown that consuming food or drink with bitter flavours is important for digestive balance and has many related health benefits.

I like Swedish Bitters, which got its name from the well-known 18th-century Swedish physician and rector of medicine Dr Claus Samst. Dr Samst rediscovered the formula through a family tradition, and he himself lived to be 104 (he finally succumbed, not to the ravages of old age, but to the result of a fall while out riding).

The actual creation of the formula is credited to Dr Phillipus Paracelsus, a Swiss physician who lived around 1541. However, it was Maria Treben, the distinguished Austrian herbalist, who brought Swedish Bitters to the world's attention.

Digestive enzymes

These are available in tablet form. Take one or two tablets right before your meal, along with your apple cider vinegar and bitters mixture. Digestive enzymes will help you fully break down those nutrients you ingest. As I explained earlier, if your stomach acid is too high, that will actually not allow you to break down the food you're eating, so you must get plenty of enzymes. It's not something you'll need to take for the rest of your life, but you can take it for a time until your stomach acid balances out.

Slippery elm

This is a demulcent herbal remedy that can soothe heartburn. Slippery elm comes in a powdered form; a gruel made by mixing one–two teaspoons of slippery elm powder with warm water can bring quick relief.

Move your body

When you're suffering from IBS, depression and anxiety, exercising is probably the last thing you feel like doing. But studies have found that even light-intensity activities, like a leisurely walk that doesn't noticeably increase your heart rate, breathing or sweating, was associated with greater psychological wellbeing and lowered rates of depression. And – cautionary tale, here – adults who were sedentary had the lowest levels of subjective wellbeing and the highest levels of depression.[19]

You don't have to exercise for hours every day, either; related findings indicate that as little as one hour of exercise each week, regardless of intensity, can help to prevent depression.[20]

Understanding (as you now do) the connection between IBS, depression and anxiety, you'll be unsurprised to learn that studies have shown that exercise also benefits your IBS. Apparently, physical activity not only keeps IBS symptoms from getting worse over time, but also actually improves the condition.

In one such study, half the participants were asked to perform moderate to vigorous physical activity for 20 to 30 minutes, three to five times a week. The other half just maintained their regular lifestyle.

Participants were asked to rate their different IBS complaints, such as abdominal pain, stool problems and quality of life. The group with unchanged lifestyles had symptoms that had become worse, by five points. But the active group showed symptom improvement of 51 points![21]

This is true, by the way, even if you're currently carrying more weight than you should. Studies show that obese people who incorporated some form of physical activity into their routine suffered less from GI symptoms than others who were inactive.[22]

Yoga and deep breathing

Studies have shown that yoga and deep breathing can be more effective for depression than drugs. And as you know by now, if it's effective for depression, it's going to help with your IBS as well! Doing yoga and deep breathing exercises just twice a week can lift major depression. With antidepressant drugs failing in half of all cases, it's an effective alternative that really does work, say the scientists.

Researchers at the Boston University Medical Center in the USA tested the yoga and deep breathing approach on a group of people diagnosed with a major depressive disorder. They discovered that the exercises 'significantly' reduced symptoms of chronic depression. Some of the subjects had never taken antidepressants, but others were still taking the drugs, even though they weren't helping.

The patients were taught Iyengar yoga, which requires precise movements and breath control. Some had two sessions a week, and others had three, but both were also asked to continue doing yoga and breath control at home on the other days.

Both groups reported a major lifting of their symptoms, although those who attended three lessons fared slightly better. Even so, two sessions had a big effect, and may be more realistic for people with busy lives, say the researchers. Yoga is a new way to treat depression, the study authors say, as it focuses on different neural pathways.[23]

Get outside and get dirty

Many of us long for 'the good life' – growing our own veg, gardening, getting our hands into the dirt, enjoying a simple return to nature. Turns out that there's science behind it: doing those things really *does* make you happy!

British researchers have discovered that bacteria found in the soil activate a group of neurons in the brain that produce our old friend serotonin. They found that treatment of mice with a 'friendly' bacteria normally found in the soil altered their behaviour in a way similar to the effect produced by antidepressant drugs. Interest in the project arose after human cancer patients being treated with the bacteria *Mycobacterium vaccae* unexpectedly reported increases in their quality of life.[24]

Dr Chris Lowry, lead author on the paper from Bristol University, said: 'These studies help us understand how the body communicates with the brain and why a healthy immune system is important for maintaining mental health. They also leave us wondering if we shouldn't all be spending more time playing in the dirt.'[25]

Scientists have also found evidence that spending time in nature provides protection against an astonishing range of diseases, including depression, diabetes, obesity, ADHD, cardiovascular disease, cancer and many more.

Why the powerful effect? After reviewing hundreds of studies examining nature's effects on health, Ming Kuo, an environment and behaviour researcher at the University of Illinois in the USA, believes the answer lies in nature's ability to *enhance the functioning of the body's immune system*.[26]

Kuo identified as many as 21 possible pathways between nature and good health – and remarked on the importance of the immune system in every one of the diseases that nature protects against. 'Nature doesn't just have one or two active ingredients,' she says. 'It's more like a multivitamin that provides us with all sorts of the nutrients we need. That's how nature can protect us from all these different kinds of diseases – cardiovascular, respiratory, mental health, musculoskeletal, etc – simultaneously.'[27]

Apparently the relationship between nature, health and the immune system is that exposure to nature switches the body into 'rest and digest' mode, which is the opposite of the 'fight or flight' mode.[28]

(Remember: when the body is in 'fight or flight mode, it shuts down everything that's immediately non-essential, including your immune system and your digestion!) When you feel completely safe – as when you're relaxing out in nature – your body feels free to devote resources to long-term projects like growing, reproducing and building the immune system.[29]

But what if you prefer indoor activities? You'll still get some of the same goodies, because being absorbed and relaxed will make your parasympathetic system happy and give your immune system a bit of a boost. However, indoors you're missing out on all the beneficial phytoncides, *Mycobacterium vaccae*, negative air ions, vitamin D-producing sunlight and other active health-boosting goodies found outdoors.[30]

So a gentle stroll outside in the fresh air, or an hour of gardening, really will do you the world of good!

Other therapies that can help

Up to this point, we've been concentrating on ways to impact the gut in order to affect the brain (as well as the gut itself). But how about turning the feedback loop around the other way, and beginning with the brain side of things?

Because of the two-way biochemical connection between the gut and the brain, we already know that the normal stress of everyday life can aggravate certain gastrointestinal conditions. This can create a vicious cycle in which worrying about or dwelling on severe pain, constipation, diarrhoea and other gastrointestinal symptoms can make the symptoms worse, which in turn increases the stress.

But if it's really true that the gut and the brain are locked into a connected feedback loop, and messing with one will always impact the other, then it should be true that working positively with the brain should help your IBS, right? And indeed, this is the case.

Hypnotherapy

Research has demonstrated that behavioural treatments specifically designed to target gut–brain pathways can be just as effective – or even more effective – than medication in helping to reduce the symptoms of IBS.

Four different studies show that hypnotherapy offers effective, lasting relief for IBS, even when the treatment isn't provided by highly specialized hypnotherapy centres. Hypnotherapy treatment improves gastrointestinal symptoms and quality of life, and patient satisfaction is very high.[31]

Cognitive behavioural therapy

Cognitive behavioural therapy (CBT) has been shown to help, as well. CBT is an umbrella term for a number of different therapies, each of which is based on the idea that thoughts, feelings, physiology and behaviour are interrelated. Treatments are designed to help people develop alternative ways of thinking and behaving, with the goal of reducing psychological distress and physiological arousal.[32]

CBT uses behavioural relaxation techniques, including diaphragmatic breathing (also known as belly breathing or deep breathing) and gut-directed hypnotherapy.[33]

It is speculated that the greater improvement observed in patients who received CBT may be due to the fact that treatments often incorporate 'exposure', a technique in which individuals gradually expose themselves to uncomfortable situations. For someone with IBS, this could include taking long road trips, eating out at restaurants and going to places where bathrooms are not readily accessible.[34]

An Epsom salts bath

Are you deficient in magnesium? Chances are good that you are – research suggests that roughly 80 per cent of us have low levels of this important mineral. If your gut has been damaged by long-term medication use, your gut bugs will struggle to absorb minerals properly, including magnesium, and you'll end up deficient.

Magnesium deficiency triggers lots of disorders, including mental illness and digestive disorders: signs of it include leg cramps, anxiety, muscle pain, weakness, fatigue, loss of appetite, apathy, confusion, insomnia, migraines, irritability, poor memory and reduced ability to learn. If you have gastrointestinal issues, you're at high risk for magnesium deficiency.

Taking a bath in Epsom salts, which contains magnesium in a form that can be absorbed through the skin, is a great solution. The chemical formula for magnesium sulfate is $MgSO4$, which shows that Epsom salts can be broken down into magnesium, sulphur and oxygen. Epsom salts is composed of small, colourless crystals and looks similar to table salt – however, table salt is completely different from Epsom salts as it consists of sodium chloride.[35]

Soaking your body, or just your feet, in a bath containing Epsom salts can increase internal levels of magnesium naturally, without the need for a supplement. An Epsom salts bath will also reduce stress, pain levels and inflammation throughout the body.[36]

According to research from the University of North Carolina in the USA, magnesium deficiency enhances stress reactions.[37] Further studies show that magnesium has a profound effect on stress and neural excitability,[38] and magnesium salts such as Epsom salts can reduce stress and improve neuropsychiatric disorders.[39] Magnesium is critical to the production of energy in cells so, by increasing magnesium levels, you can feel revived without feeling restless (as opposed to how people feel revived from caffeine consumption).[40]

An Epsom salts bath will also draw the toxins out of your body, helping to get rid of the bad bugs that the kefir is purging from your system – it's a great 'pull' technology to help with your detox while following the Kefir Solution.

How to take your Epsom salts bath

Add 250g/10oz Epsom salts to bathwater and soak for 40 minutes maximum. The first 20 minutes gives your body time to remove toxins from your system, while the last 20 minutes will allow you to absorb the minerals in the water and help you emerge from the bath feeling rejuvenated.[41]

For a foot bath, add 125g/5oz Epsom salts to a large pan of warm water and soak your feet for 20 minutes. Be sure to drink water before, during and after both the full-body and foot baths, to protect yourself from dehydration and increase detoxification.[42]

Unlike other salts, external contact with Epsom salts doesn't make the skin feel dry: it leaves it feeling soft and silky.

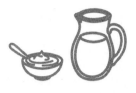

Conclusion

I hope that by now you understand yourself, your gut bugs, and the connection between your gut and your brain more clearly. I hope that you can see what a marvellous constellation of little life forms, all hooked together into a sophisticated, delicate, interconnected ecosystem, you really are!

I hope that you can see how this fragile holobiont can be damaged through the misuse of sugar and antibiotics. Even more importantly, I hope that you now understand how to repair that damage by working with the natural healing properties of kefir, ashwagandha, your feelings, your food, and changes to your lifestyle.

Given time and some discipline, the Kefir Solution *will* help to resolve your IBS, depression and anxiety: and it may also help you in other ways that both surprise and delight you. As your microbiome recovers its health and vigour, your system will begin to sing again – like a plant that's finally being watered.

Please keep me posted on your progress – I dearly love to receive updates from fellow travellers on this journey! I'm here if you need me. You can contact me through my website: www.chucklinggoat. co.uk.

I'd like to leave you with two thoughts, before we finish.

You are the expert of your own wellness

No one is inside your skin, except you. No expert can tell you – or predict – how your particular microbiome will react to a certain food. Your gut microbiome began with a unique genetic inheritance from your parents, and has since undergone specific stresses and strains through the years, driving the population in a particular way. At this moment, your microbiome is as individual to you as your fingerprint.

It's oh-so-tempting to turn this process over to the smart people in the white coats, and ask them to tell us what we can and cannot eat. I've given you some suggestions in this book, based on the science that's out there, but only *you* can truly determine what, how much, when and which foods to consume.

So, how are you going to figure it out? Let me offer you one of my favourite concepts, which I learned in the study of medical herbs: *organoleptic*. Great word, right? It means *acting on, or involving the use of, the sense organs.*

Conduct an *organoleptic search* to see which foods you need to be consuming. Wake up your senses – how does a particular food smell to you? We get a huge amount of information through our olfactory senses, and your gut bugs are in close communication with your brain, feeding back information about whether or not a food would be beneficial.

Touch the food. How does it feel between your fingers? Take a pinch and put it on your tongue. Close your eyes, and pay attention to the minute reactions of your body. Chew it. Swallow it. How does it feel now? Wait 10 minutes, then 20. Now what's going on? Take notes. Write everything down, so that you can refer to your impressions later.

In fact, all the way through your Kefir Solution journey, I recommend that you take detailed notes, with dates and responses: so that you can create your own case study, and your own metrics. This will not only help you keep track of the progress you make over time, but will also make your GP or consultant take you much more seriously.

The organoleptic process is the way that humans learned which foods were safe for them to consume, long before people wrote books to tell them what to do. You have millions of years' worth of organoleptic knowledge encoded in your DNA – you're wiser than you know. Wake up your intuition, and listen to it! It will give you all the information you need in order to proceed.

The Kefir Solution is not complicated

There's a good reason for this: *you're a part of nature.* Your body works according to natural principles (a principle is something that's fundamentally true, wherever it's applied). These principles are always the same, wherever you look, and they work for whatever you're taking care of.

In many ways, healing your gut–brain connection is like an ecological restoration project. Imagine poor soil, important species missing from the ecosystem, healthy cycles broken. You can restore the health of your own system in exactly the same way you'd repair a devastated landscape in nature.

First, you bring in pioneer organisms that suppress weeds and support healthy growth: that's the kefir. Then you promote and support biodiversity in the system. And celebrate as it slowly begins to bloom again!

Whether it's a baby, an animal, your own inner gut bugs or the planetary ecosystem around you, the rules for nurturing something are the same, and they are simpler

- Love it.

- Feed it.

- Don't poison it.

Look after your internal ecosystem, in the same way you look after your family; in the same way you look after the global ecosystem outside. Look after the world around you, in the same way you look after yourself. We are all connected.

Remember: there are as many tiny life forms inside you as there are observable stars in the universe.

You are the planet.

Let it shine.

Hugs from the barn,

Shann x

References

Introduction

1. Technische Universitaet Muenchen. 'Proof that a gut-wrenching complaint – irritable bowel syndrome – is not in your head.' ScienceDaily. *ScienceDaily*, 20 August 2010. <www.sciencedaily.com/releases/2010/08/100819141950.htm>.

2. Mayo Clinic. 'Irritable bowel syndrome definitely isn't "all in the head". ScienceDaily. *ScienceDaily*, 13 November 2012. <www.sciencedaily.com/releases/2012/11/121113122135.htm>.

3. Mayo Clinic. 'Genetic clue to irritable bowel syndrome found.' ScienceDaily. *ScienceDaily*, 20 March 2014. <www.sciencedaily.com/releases/2014/03/140320173158.htm>.

4. American Gastroenterological Association. 'IBS and bloating: When gut microbiota gets out of balance.' ScienceDaily. *ScienceDaily*, 10 March 2014. <www.sciencedaily.com/releases/2014/03/140310090921.htm>.

5. American College of Gastroenterology. 'Psychological traumas experienced over lifetime linked to adult irritable bowel syndrome.' ScienceDaily. *ScienceDaily*, 5 November 2011. <www.sciencedaily.com/releases/2011/10/111031115101.htm>.

Chapter 1: Meet Your Microbiome

1. American Gastroenterological Association. 'IBS and bloating: When gut microbiota gets out of balance.' ScienceDaily. *ScienceDaily*, 10 March 2014. <www.sciencedaily.com/releases/2014/03/140310090921.htm>.

2. Cell Press. 'Gut microbe movements regulate host circadian rhythms.' ScienceDaily. *ScienceDaily*, 1 December 2016. <www.sciencedaily.com/releases/2016/12/161201121135.htm>.

3. Ibid.

4. American Physiological Society (APS). 'Food and antibiotics may change microorganisms in gut, causing IBS.' ScienceDaily. *ScienceDaily*, 26 January 2017. <www.sciencedaily.com/releases/2017/01/170126120109.htm>.

5. Oregon State University. 'Common antimicrobial agent rapidly disrupts gut bacteria.' ScienceDaily. *ScienceDaily*, 18 May 2016. <www.sciencedaily.com/releases/2016/05/160518152805.htm>.

Chapter 2: The Connection Between Anxiety, Depression and IBS

1. VIB – Flanders Interuniversity Institute for Biotechnology. 'Anxiety increases risk of gastrointestinal infection, long-term complications.' ScienceDaily. *ScienceDaily*, 2 July 2015. <www.sciencedaily.com/releases/2015/07/150702073929.htm>.

2. American College of Gastroenterology. 'Psychological traumas experienced over lifetime linked to adult irritable bowel syndrome.' ScienceDaily. *ScienceDaily*, 5 November 2011. <www.sciencedaily.com/releases/2011/10/111031115101.htm>.

3. Zhou Linghong. 'Psychobiotics and the gut–brain axis: in the pursuit of happiness.' *Neuropsychiatric Disease and Treatment*. 16 March 2015. <www.ncbi.nlm.nih.gov/pmc/articles/PMC4370913/>.

4. Cedars-Sinai Medical Center. 'Irritable bowel syndrome clearly linked to gut bacteria.' ScienceDaily. *ScienceDaily*, 25 May 2012. <www.sciencedaily.com/releases/2012/05/120525103354.htm>.

5. McMaster University. 'Intestinal bacteria alter gut and brain function, study shows.' ScienceDaily. *ScienceDaily*, 1 March 2017. <www.sciencedaily.com/releases/2017/03/170301142503.htm>.

6. Wiley. 'Gastrointestinal disorders involve both brain-to-gut and gut-to-brain pathways.' ScienceDaily. *ScienceDaily*, 22 July 2016. <www.sciencedaily.com/releases/2016/07/160722093247.htm>.

7. BioMed Central. 'High Risk Of Migraine, Depression And Chronic Pain For IBS Sufferers, Large Study Shows.' ScienceDaily. *ScienceDaily*, 28 September 2006. <www.sciencedaily.com/releases/2006/09/060928095529.htm>.

8. Wiley. 'Gastrointestinal disorders involve both brain-to-gut and gut-to-brain pathways.' ScienceDaily. *ScienceDaily*, 22 July 2016. <www.sciencedaily.com/releases/2016/07/160722093247.htm>.

9. Mayo Clinic. 'St. John's wort not helpful treatment for irritable bowel syndrome, researchers say.' ScienceDaily. *ScienceDaily*, 5 January 2010. <www.sciencedaily.com/releases/2010/01/100104114559.htm>.

10. Loyola University Health System. 'Health psychologists now treating functional heartburn, Crohn's Disease, IBS and other GI disorders.' ScienceDaily. *ScienceDaily*, 23 March 2017. <www.sciencedaily.com/releases/2017/03/170323141632.htm>.

11. Medical University of Vienna. 'Depression detectable in the blood: Platelet serotonin transporter function.' ScienceDaily. *ScienceDaily*, 29 April 2014. <www.sciencedaily.com/releases/2014/04/140429105015.htm>.

12. Chicago Rush University Medical Center. 'Allergic Disease Linked To Irritable Bowel Syndrome.' ScienceDaily. *ScienceDaily*, 31 January 2008. <www.sciencedaily.com/releases/2008/01/080130170325.htm>.

13. University of California, Los Angeles. 'Brain Response Differences In The Way Women With IBS Anticipate And React To Pain.' ScienceDaily. *ScienceDaily*, 12 January 2008. <www.sciencedaily.com/releases/2008/01/080108183122.htm>.

14. United European Gastroenterology. 'Link between depression, abnormal brain response to visceral pain in patients with IBS.' ScienceDaily. *ScienceDaily*, 2 October 2014. <www.sciencedaily.com/releases/2014/10/141002123641.htm>.

15. University of California, Los Angeles. 'Structural brain alterations in patients with irritable bowel syndrome discovered.' ScienceDaily. *ScienceDaily*, 23 July 2010. <www.sciencedaily.com/releases/2010/07/100722132433.htm>.

16. University of Exeter. 'Gut microorganisms affect our physiology.' ScienceDaily. *ScienceDaily*, 29 December 2016. < University of Exeter. 'Gut microorganisms affect our physiology>

17. Alimentary Pharmabiotic Centre, University College Cork. 'Early gut bacteria regulate happiness.' ScienceDaily. *ScienceDaily*, 12 June 2012. <www.sciencedaily.com/releases/2012/06/120612115812.htm>.

18. American Gastroenterological Association. 'Effectiveness Of Serotonin And Nerve Stimulants On Irritable Bowel Syndromes Evaluated.' ScienceDaily. *ScienceDaily*, 24 May 2007. <www.sciencedaily.com/releases/2007/05/070522073647.htm>.

19. McMaster University. 'Intestinal bacteria alter gut and brain function, study shows.' ScienceDaily. *ScienceDaily*, 1 March 2017. <www. sciencedaily.com/releases/2017/03/170301142503.htm>.

Chapter 3: What's the Big Deal about Serotonin?

1. Oregon Health & Science University. 'Researchers visualize brain's serotonin pump, provide blueprint for new, more effective SSRIs: Revealing serotonin transporter's molecular structure opens new era of drug treatments for depression and anxiety.' ScienceDaily. *ScienceDaily*, 6 April 2016. <https://www.sciencedaily.com/releases/2016/04/160406140336.htm>

2. UCSF Benioff Children's Hospital Oakland. 'Omega-3 fatty acids, vitamin D may control brain serotonin, affecting behavior and psychiatric disorders.' ScienceDaily. *ScienceDaily*, 25 February 2015. <www.sciencedaily.com/releases/2015/02/150225094109.htm>.

3. American Gastroenterological Association. 'Effectiveness Of Serotonin And Nerve Stimulants On Irritable Bowel Syndromes Evaluated.' ScienceDaily. *ScienceDaily*, 24 May 2007. <www.sciencedaily.com/releases/2007/05/070522073647.htm>.

4. University of Southern California. 'Critical role of placenta in brain development demonstrated.' ScienceDaily. *ScienceDaily*, 22 April 2011. <www.sciencedaily.com/releases/2011/04/110421104516.htm>.

5. Columbia University Medical Center. 'It Takes Guts To Build Bone, Scientists Discover.' ScienceDaily. *ScienceDaily*, 1 December 2008. <www.sciencedaily.com/releases/2008/11/081126122209.htm>.

6. Elsevier Health Sciences. 'Serotonin deficiency implicated in rheumatoid arthritis: Ra symptoms and pathology worse in mice missing enzyme needed for serotonin synthesis.' ScienceDaily. *ScienceDaily*, 9 March 2016. <www.sciencedaily.com/releases/2016/03/160309140034.htm>.

7. Johns Hopkins Medicine. 'Brain scan study adds to evidence that lower brain serotonin levels are linked to dementia: Results suggest serotonin loss may be a key player in cognitive decline, not just a side-effect of Alzheimer's disease.' ScienceDaily. *ScienceDaily*, 14 August 2017. <www.sciencedaily.com/releases/2017/08/170814092943.htm>.

8. Buck Institute for Age Research. 'Serotonin receptor is involved in eczema and other itch conditions: Research points to new target for treatments.' ScienceDaily. *ScienceDaily*, 11 June 2015. <www.sciencedaily.com/releases/2015/06/150611122953.htm>.

9. University of Washington. 'Mother-daughter Conflict, Low Serotonin Level May Be Deadly Combination.' ScienceDaily. *ScienceDaily*, 7 March 2008. <www.sciencedaily.com/releases/2008/03/080305144202. htm>.

10. University of Pittsburgh Medical Center. 'Serotonin May Play Role In Hardening of the Arteries.' ScienceDaily. *ScienceDaily*, 4 March 2006. <www.sciencedaily.com/releases/2006/03/060303205220.htm>.

11. University of Cambridge. 'Serotonin levels affect the brain's response to anger.' ScienceDaily. *ScienceDaily*, 15 September 2011. <www. sciencedaily.com/releases/2011/09/110915102917.htm>.

12. University of Tsukuba. 'Tantrums, transmitters and treatments: Neurotransmitters linked aggressive behavior.' ScienceDaily. *ScienceDaily*, 23 April 2015. <www.sciencedaily.com/ releases/2015/04/150423085137.htm>.

13. Centre for Addiction and Mental Health. 'Fluctuations In Serotonin Transport May Explain Winter Blues.' ScienceDaily. *ScienceDaily*, 9 September 2008. <www.sciencedaily.com/ releases/2008/09/080908101620.htm>.

14. Karolinska Institutet. 'Sex Differences In The Brain's Serotonin System.' ScienceDaily. *ScienceDaily*, 17 February 2008. <www. sciencedaily.com/releases/2008/02/080213111043.htm>.

15. University of Zurich. 'LSD alters perception via serotonin receptors.' ScienceDaily. *ScienceDaily*, 26 January 2017. <www.sciencedaily.com/ releases/2017/01/170126123127.htm>.

16. University of California, San Francisco. 'Rare cells are "window into the gut" for the nervous system: Cells that alert nervous system to intestinal trouble could provide new target for gastrointestinal treatments.' ScienceDaily. *ScienceDaily*, 22 June 2017. <www. sciencedaily.com/releases/2017/06/170622121916.htm>.

17. Hadhazy, Adam. 'Think Twice: How the Gut's Second Brain Influence Mood and Well-Being.' *Scientific American*. 12 February 2010. <www. scientificamerican.com/article/gut-second-brain/>.

18. Public Library of Science. '45 years on: How serotonin makes schistosome parasites move.' ScienceDaily. *ScienceDaily*, 16 January 2014. <www.sciencedaily.com/releases/2014/01/140116190313.htm>.

19. Paddock, Catharine. 'Gut microbes important for serotonin production.' *Medical News Today*, 21 April 2015. <www.medicalnewstoday.com/ articles/292693.php?bl>.

20. University of Maryland Medical Center. 'Depression stems from miscommunication between brain cells; Study challenges role of serotonin in depression.' ScienceDaily. *ScienceDaily*, 18 March 2013. www.sciencedaily.com/releases/2013/03/130318105329.htm

21. The Zuckerman Institute at Columbia University. 'Neurons' faulty wiring leads to serotonin imbalance, depression-like behavior in mice: Twin papers lend clues into how the brain organizes itself, offering new avenues for studying psychiatric disorders.' ScienceDaily. *ScienceDaily*, 27 April 2017. <www.sciencedaily.com/releases/2017/04/170427141736.htm>.

22. Carasi, P. 'Impact of Kefir Derived Lactobacillus kefiri on the Mucosal Immune Response and Gut Microbiota.' *Journal of Immunology Research*. 24 February 2015. <www.ncbi.nlm.nih.gov/pmc/articles/PMC4355334/>.

23. Manocha, M. 'IL-13-mediated immunological control of enterochromaffin cell hyperplasia and serotonin production in the gut.' *Mucosal Immunology* (2013) 6, 146–155; doi:10.1038/mi.2012.58; published online 4 July 2012. </www.nature.com/mi/journal/v6/n1/full/mi201258a.html?foxtrotcallback=true>.

24. Adiloğlu, A.K. 'The effect of kefir consumption on human immune system: a cytokine study.' *Microbiology Bulletin*. 2013 Apr; 47(2):273–81. <www.ncbi.nlm.nih.gov/pubmed/23621727>.

25. University of Exeter. 'Gut microorganisms affect our physiology.' ScienceDaily. *ScienceDaily*, 29 December 2016. <www.sciencedaily.com/releases/2016/12/161229141847.htm>.

26. American Gastroenterological Association. 'Effectiveness Of Serotonin And Nerve Stimulants On Irritable Bowel Syndromes Evaluated.' ScienceDaily. *ScienceDaily*, 24 May 2007. <www.sciencedaily.com/releases/2007/05/070522073647.htm>.

27. Center for the Advancement of Health. 'Depletion Of Body Chemical Can Cause Memory, Mood Changes.' ScienceDaily. *ScienceDaily*, 19 November 2002. <www.sciencedaily.com/releases/2002/11/021119073229.htm>.

28. Institute of Molecular Biotechnology. 'How malnutrition leads to inflamed intestines.' ScienceDaily. *ScienceDaily*, 25 July 2012. <www.sciencedaily.com/releases/2012/07/120725132133.htm>.

Chapter 4: Psychobiotics – is That Really a Thing?

1. Cell Press. 'The current state of psychobiotics.' ScienceDaily. *ScienceDaily*, 25 October 2016. <www.sciencedaily.com/releases/2016/10/161025220959.htm>.

2. Dinan, T.G. 'Psychobiotics: a novel class of psychotropic.' *Biological Psychiatry.* 15 November 2013. <www.ncbi.nlm.nih.gov/pubmed/23759244>.

3. Tillish, K. 'Consumption of fermented milk product with probiotic modulates brain activity.' *Gastroenterology*, June 2013. <www.ncbi.nlm.nih.gov/pubmed/23474283>.

4. Wall, R. 'Bacterial neuroactive compounds produced by psychobiotics.' *Advances in Experimental Medicine and Biology*, 2014. <www.ncbi.nlm.nih.gov/pubmed/24997036>.

5. Ait-Belgnaoui, A. 'Probiotic gut effect prevents the chronic psychological stress-induced brain activity abnormality in mice.' *Neurogastroenterology and motility: the official journal of the European gastrointestinal Motility Society*, April 2014. <ww.ncbi.nlm.nih.gov/pubmed/24372793>.

6. Watson, S. 'HPA axis function in mood disorders.' *Science Direct.* 1 May 2006. <www.sciencedirect.com/science/article/pii/S1476179306700374>.

7. Petra, A. 'Gut-Microbiota-Brain Axis and Its Effect on Neuropsychiatric Disorders With Suspected Immune Dysregulation.' *Clinical Therapeutics*, May 2015. <www.ncbi.nlm.nih.gov/pubmed/26046241>.

8. Venket Rao, A. 'A randomized, double-blind, placebo-controlled pilot study of a probiotic in emotional symptoms of chronic fatigue syndrome.' *Gut Pathogens*, 19 March 2009. <www.gutpathogens.biomedcentral.com/articles/10.1186/1757-4749-1-6>.

9. Kato Kataoka, A. 'Fermented milk containing Lactobacillus casei strain Shirota prevents the onset of physical symptoms in medical students under academic examination stress.' *Beneficial Microbes*, 21 December 2015. <www.ncbi.nlm.nih.gov/pubmed/26689231>.

10. Zhou, Linghong. 'Psychobiotics and the gut–brain axis: in the pursuit of happiness.' *Neuroosychiatric Disease and Treatment*, 16 March 2015. <www.ncbi.nlm.nih.gov/pmc/articles/PMC4370913/>.

11. American College of Gastroenterology. 'How Effective Are Probiotics In Irritable Bowel Syndrome?' ScienceDaily. *ScienceDaily*, 10 October 2008. <www.sciencedaily.com/releases/2008/10/081006092656.htm>.

12. McMaster University. 'Probiotic use linked to improved symptoms of depression.' ScienceDaily. *ScienceDaily*, 23 May 2017. <www.sciencedaily.com/releases/2017/05/170523124119.htm>.

13. Liang, S. 'Administration of Lactobacillus helveticus NS8 improves behavioral, cognitive, and biochemical aberrations caused by chronic restraint stress.' *Neuroscience*, 3 December 2015. <www.ncbi.nlm.nih.gov/pubmed/26408987>.

14. Office of Naval Research. 'Gut feeling: Research examines link between stomach bacteria, PTSD.' ScienceDaily. *ScienceDaily*, 25 April 2016. <www.sciencedaily.com/releases/2016/04/160425161324.htm>.

Chapter 6: The Kefir Solution Step #1: Drink Kefir

1. BBC News. Health. 'Which foods can improve your gut bacteria?' 30 January 2017. </www.bbc.co.uk/news/health-38800977>.

2. Ibid.

3. BBC News. Health. 'Which foods can improve your gut bacteria?' 30 January 2017. </www.bbc.co.uk/news/health-38800977>.

4. American Society for Microbiology. 'Dairy products boost effectiveness of probiotics.' ScienceDaily. *ScienceDaily*, 17 July 2015. <www.sciencedaily.com/releases/2015/07/150717142439.htm>.

5. Canadian Science Publishing (NRC Research Press). 'Potent protein heals wounds, boosts immunity and protects from cancer.' ScienceDaily. *ScienceDaily*, 30 April 2012. <www.sciencedaily.com/releases/2012/04/120430164353.htm>.

6. Axe, Josh. 'Goat Milk Benefits Are Superior to Cow Milk.' *Food Is Medicine*. <draxe.com/goat-milk/>.

7. University of Granada. 'Goats' Milk Is More Beneficial To Health Than Cows' Milk, Study Suggests.' ScienceDaily. *ScienceDaily*, 31 July 2007. <www.sciencedaily.com/releases/2007/07/070730100229.htm>.

8. Kresser, Chris. '3 reasons why coconut milk may not be your friend. Let's take back your health, starting now.' 9 June 2011. <chriskresser.com/3-reasons-why-coconut-milk-may-not-be-your-friend/>.

9. Soy Alert! Studies showing adverse effects of soy: https://www.westonaprice.org/soy-alert/

10. Marco, Mariángeles Briggiler. 'Bacteriophages and dairy fermentations.' Published by Journal List, 1 July 2012. ncbi.nlm.nih.gov/pmc/articles/PMC3530524

11. Norwegian School of Veterinary Science. 'Viruses can turn Harmless E.Coli dangerous.' Published by ScienceDaily on 22 April 2009. sciencedaily.com/releases/2009/04/090417195827.htm

12. Stanford University Medical Center. 'Tryptophan No Turkey In Boosting Immune System, Stanford Study Shows.' ScienceDaily. *ScienceDaily*, 9 November 2005. <www.sciencedaily.com/releases/2005/11/051107082352.htm>.

Chapter 7: The Kefir Solution Step #2: Take Ashwagandha

1. Borreli, Lizette. 'What's The Best Time To Drink Coffee? The Hour Matters Because Cortisol Cycle Influences Caffeine Effectiveness.' *Medical Daily*. 8 Nov 2013. <www.medicaldaily.com/whats-best-time-drink-coffee-hour-matters-because-cortisol-cycle-influences-caffeine-effectiveness>.

2. Schalinski, I. et al. 'The Cortisol Paradox of Trauma-Related Disorders: Lower Phasic Responses But Higher Tonic Levels of Cortisol are Associated with Sexual Abuse in Childhood.' *PLoS One* 10 e0136921 (2015).

3. 'Chronic Stress Puts Your Health At Risk.' Stress Management, Mayo Clinic, <www.mayoclinic.org/healthy-lifestyle/stress-management/in-depth/stress/art-20046037>.

4. Chandrasekhar, K. et al. 'A prospective, randomized double-blind, placebo-controlled study of safety and efficacy of a high-concentration full-spectrum extract of ashwagandha root in reducing stress and anxiety in adults.' *Indian Journal of Psychological Medicine* 34, no. 3 (2012): 255. <www.ncbi.nlm.nih.gov/pmc/articles/PMC3573577/>.

5. Ibid.

6. Bhattacharya, S.K. Anxiolytic-antidepressant activity of Withania somnifera glycowithanolides: an experimental study.' *Phytomedicine*. Dec 2000; 7(6):463-9. <www.ncbi.nlm.nih.gov/pubmed/11194174>.

7. Umadevi, M. 'Traditional and medicinal uses of Withania somnifera.' *The Pharma Innovation* 1, no. 9 (2012).

8. Cooley, K. et al. 'Naturopathic care for anxiety: a randomized controlled trial ISRCTN78958974.' *PLoS One* 4, no. 8 (2009): e6628.

9. Chandrasekhar, K. et al. 'A prospective, randomized double-blind, placebo-controlled study of safety and efficacy of a high-concentration full-spectrum extract of ashwagandha root in reducing stress and anxiety in adults.' *Indian Journal of Psychological Medicine* 34, no. 3 (2012): 255. <www.ncbi.nlm.nih.gov/pmc/articles/PMC3573577/>.

10. Chittaranjan, A. et al. 'A double-blind, placebo-controlled evaluation of the anxiolytic efficacy of an ethanolic extract of withania somnifera.' *Indian Journal of Psychiatry* 42, no. 3 (2000): 295.

11. Axe, Josh. 'Ashwagandha Benefits Thyroid and Adrenals.' *Dr Axe Food Is Medicine.* <www.draxe.com/ashwagandha-proven-to-heal-thyroid-and-adrenals/>.

Chapter 8: The Kefir Solution Step #3: Lean in to Your Feelings

1. Whiteman, Honor. 'Embracing negative emotions could boost psychological well-being.' *Medical News Today.* 13 August 2017. <www.medicalnewstoday.com/articles/318933.php>.

2. Ibid.

3. Baer, Drake. 'How Only Being Able to Use Logic to Make Decisions Destroyed a Man's Life.' Science of Us. *New York Magazine*, 14 June 2016. <nymag.com/scienceofus/2016/06/how-only-using-logic-destroyed-a-man.html>.

4. <http://articles.mercola.com/sites/articles/archive/2017/08/16/remedies-to-prevent-dry-eyes.aspx?utm_source=dnl&utm_medium=email&utm_content=art2&utm_campaign=20170816Z2&et_cid=DM154648&et_rid=16723864>.

5. Ibid.

6. <https://articles.mercola.com/sites/articles/archive/2017/09/10/processed-foods-health-effects.aspx>.

7. Ibid.

8. <https://articles.mercola.com/sites/articles/archive/2017/09/10/processed-foods-health-effects.aspx>.

9. Lustig, Robert H. *The Hacking of the American Mind: The Science Behind the Corporate Takeover of Our Bodies and Brains.* Avery, Penguin Random House. 2017.

10. https://articles.mercola.com/sites/articles/archive/2017/09/10/processed-foods-health-effects.aspx

11. Lustig, Robert H. *The Hacking of the American Mind: The Science Behind the Corporate Takeover of Our Bodies and Brains.* Avery, Penguin Random House. 2017.

12. Ibid.

Chapter 9: The Kefir Solution Step #4: Alter Your Eating Habits

1. *Daily Mail.* 'Women have tried 61 diets by the age of 45 in the constant battle to stay slim.' 20 March 2012. <www.dailymail.co.uk/health/article-2117445/Women-tried-61-diets-age-45-constant-battle-stay-slim.html#ixzz4yIDu33JA>.

2. University of California, Los Angeles, Health Sciences. 'Changing gut bacteria through diet affects brain function.' ScienceDaily. *ScienceDaily*, 28 May 2013. <www.sciencedaily.com/releases/2013/05/130528180900.htm>.

3. Ibid.

4. Arizona State University. 'War and peace in the human gut: Probing the microbiome.' ScienceDaily. *ScienceDaily*, 6 June 2016. <www.sciencedaily.com/releases/2016/06/160606200431.htm>.

5. Ibid.

6. Washington University School of Medicine. 'Protein-rich diet may help soothe inflamed gut: Mice fed tryptophan develop immune cells that foster a tolerant gut.' ScienceDaily. *ScienceDaily*, 3 August 2017. <www.sciencedaily.com/releases/2017/08/170803141045.htm>.

7. Chow, Janet, et al. 'Getting the Bugs out of the Immune System: Do Bacterial Microbiota "Fix" Intestinal T Cell Responses?' *Cell Host & Microbe*. Volume 5, Issue 1, 22 January 2009, Pages 8-12. </www.sciencedirect.com/science/article/pii/S193131280800406X>.

8. Washington University School of Medicine. 'Protein-rich diet may help soothe inflamed gut: Mice fed tryptophan develop immune cells that foster a tolerant gut.' ScienceDaily. *ScienceDaily*, 3 August 2017. <www.sciencedaily.com/releases/2017/08/170803141045.htm>.

Chapter 10: The Kefir Solution Eating Principles

1. Leiden, Universiteit. 'Trust through food.' ScienceDaily. *ScienceDaily*, 22 October 2013. <www.sciencedaily.com/releases/2013/10/131022101930.htm>.

2. AMA and Archives Journals. 'Compounds in non-stick cookware may be associated with elevated cholesterol in children and teens.' ScienceDaily. *ScienceDaily*, 7 September 2010. <sciencedaily.com/releases/2010/09/100906203040.htm>.

3. Egan, Hope. 'Ten Reasons to Try Cast-Iron Cooking.' *Natural News*, 18 March 2011. <www. naturalnews.com/031737_cast_iron_cookware.html>.

4. University of Eastern Filllaild. Illgh chrlootorol diet eating eggs do not increase risk of heart attack, not even in persons genetically predisposed, study finds.' ScienceDaily. *ScienceDaily*, 11 February 2016. <www.sciencedaily.com/releases/2016/02/160211083044.htm>.

5. University of Alberta. 'Eggs' antioxidant properties may help prevent heart disease and cancer, study suggests.' ScienceDaily. *ScienceDaily*, 6 July 2011. <www.sciencedaily.com/releases/2011/07/110706093900.htm>.

6. Allen, Jeffrey A. 'Post-epidemic eosinophilia myalgia syndrome associated with L-Tryptophan.' *Arthritis Rheum*. November 2011; 63(11): 10.1002/art.30514. doi: 10.1002/art.30514. <www.ncbi.nlm. nih.gov/pmc/articles/PMC3848710/>.

7. Office of Naval Research. 'Gut feeling: Research examines link between stomach bacteria, PTSD.' ScienceDaily. *ScienceDaily*, 25 April 2016. <www.sciencedaily.com/releases/2016/04/160425161324.htm>.

8. European Academy of Neurology. 'Connections between gut microbiota and the brain.' ScienceDaily. *ScienceDaily*, 29 May 2016. <www.sciencedaily.com/releases/2016/05/160529174445.htm>.

9. Bourrie, Benjamin. 'The Microbiota and Health Promoting Characteristics of the Fermented Beverage Kefir.' *Frontiers in Microbiology*, 4 May 2016. <www.ncbi.nlm.nih.gov/pmc/articles/PMC4854945/>.

10. Cell Press. 'How humans and their gut microbes may respond to plant hormones.' ScienceDaily. *ScienceDaily*, 22 August 2017. <www.sciencedaily.com/releases/2017/08/170822123844.htm>.

11. American Association for Cancer Research. 'Eating resistant starch may help reduce red meat-related colorectal cancer risk.' ScienceDaily. *ScienceDaily*, 4 August 2014. <www.sciencedaily.com/releases/2014/08/140804100346.htm>.

12. University of Colorado Denver. 'Diet of resistant starch helps the body resist colorectal cancer'. ScienceDaily. *ScienceDaily*, 19 February 2013. <www.sciencedaily.com/releases/2013/02/130219140716.htm>.

13. Society of Chemical Industry. 'Potato Salad May Help the Immune System.' ScienceDaily. *ScienceDaily*, 25 June 2007. <www.sciencedaily.com/releases/2007/06/070625080937.htm>.

14. American Association for Cancer Research. 'Eating resistant starch may help reduce red meat-related colorectal cancer risk'. ScienceDaily. *ScienceDaily*, 4 August 2014. <www.sciencedaily.com/ releases/2014/08/140804100346.htm>.

15. University of Illinois at Urbana-Champaign. 'Legumes Found To Contain Starch Carrying A Fiber-Like Punch.' ScienceDaily. *ScienceDaily*, 7 February 2001. <www.sciencedaily.com/ releases/2001/02/010205080131.htm>.

16. University of Colorado Denver. 'Diet of resistant starch helps the body resist colorectal cancer.' ScienceDaily. *ScienceDaily*, 19 February 2013. <www.sciencedaily.com/releases/2013/02/130219140716.htm>.

17. Semeco, Arlene. 'Seven Health Benefits of Psyllium.' *Medical News Today*. 31 July 2017. <www.medicalnewstoday.com/articles/318707. php>.

18. Shivanna, N. 'Antioxidant, anti-diabetic and renal protective properties of Stevia rebaudiana.' Elsevier Inc., 7 November 2012. <www.ncbi.nlm.nih.gov/pubmed/23140911>.

19. Goyal, S.K. 'Stevia (Stevia rebaudiana) a bio-sweetener: a review.' Taylor & Francis, 13 February 2010. <www.ncbi.nlm.nih.gov/ pubmed/19961353>.

20. Verburgh, Kris. *The Food Hourglass*. HarperCollins, 2014.

21. Whiteman, Honor. 'Too much sugar may harm men's mental health' *Medical News Today*. 28 July 2017. <www.medicalnewstoday.com/ articles/318692.php>.

22. NHS Choices. 'Can Honey Fight Superbugs like MRSA'. NHS, 13 April 2011. <www.nhs.uk/news/2011/04April/Pages/manuka-honey-mrsa-superbug-bacteria.aspx>.

23. Morgan, Maybelle. 'Is your superfood honey fake? Experts reveal that three times more jars of healing manuka are sold around the world than being produced in New Zealand'. *Daily Mail* 3 May 2015. <www.dailymail.co.uk/femail/article-3066381/Is-superfood-honey-FAKE-jars-manuka-sold-world-produced-New-Zealand.html>.

24. *Daily Mail* reporter. 'Scottish honey 'is as good at healing as manuka': Heather variety could offer cheaper alternative.' *Daily Mail*, 2 October 2013. <www.dailymail.co.uk/health/article-2440926/Scottish-honey-good-healing-manuka-Heather-variety-offer-cheaper-alternative.html#ixzz4AiVVJXiU>.

25. Spector, Tim. 'My dad asked me to eat McDonald's for 10 days. This is what happened.' *The Telegraph*, 14 May 2015. <www.telegraph.co.uk/foodanddrink/11603430/My-dad-made-me-eat-McDonalds for 10 days -This-is-what-happened.html>.

26. Thomas, James. 'Milk Allergy May Be Masquerading As Milk Intolerance In Some Adults'. Health Central, 2 April 2013. <www.healthcentral.com/allergy/c/3989/160106/milk-masquerading-intolerance>.

27. El-Agamy, E.I. 'The challenge of cow milk protein allergy.' Science Direct. *Small Ruminant Research* 68 (2007) 64–72. 20 October 2006. <www.camelnet.eu/wp-content/uploads/2014/09/thechallenge ofcowmilkproteinallergy.pdf>.

28. University of Granada. 'Goat milk can be considered as functional food, Spanish researchers find.' ScienceDaily. *ScienceDaily*, 20 May 2011. <www.sciencedaily.com/releases/2011/05/110518092146. htm>.

29. Ibid.

30. Ibid.

31. Ibid.

Chapter 11: The Kefir Solution Eating Plan

1. https://www.ncbi.nlm.nih.gov/pubmed/21631511

2. http://psychologyofeating.com/metabolic-power-pleasure/

3. American Chemical Society. 'Benefits of nut consumption for people with abdominal obesity, high blood sugar, high blood pressure.' ScienceDaily. *ScienceDaily*, 10 November 2011. <www.sciencedaily. com/releases/2011/11/111102125348.htm>.

4. Universidad de Barcelona. 'Study suggests new benefits of eating nuts for patients with metabolic syndrome.' ScienceDaily. *ScienceDaily*, 12 November 2011. <www.sciencedaily.com/ releases/2011/11/111111095222.htm>.

5. Wilson, Sarah. 'How to Live to 100: eat pork.' 7 August 2012. <www. sarahwilson.com/2012/08/how-to-live-to-100-eat-pork/>.

6. University of Cambridge. 'Serotonin Link To Impulsivity, Decision-making, Confirmed.' ScienceDaily. *ScienceDaily*, 11 June 2008. <www. sciencedaily.com/releases/2008/06/080605150908.htm>.

7. 'Chocolate Is The Most Widely Craved Food, But Is It Really Addictive?' ScienceDaily. *ScienceDaily*, 12 September 2007. <www.sciencedaily.com/releases/2007/09/070911073921.htm>.

8. Bushak, Lecia. 'Wine and Coffee May Be Good for Your Gut Bacteria, Helping to Diversifiy Your Microbiome.' *Medical Daily*. 29 April 2016. <www.medicaldaily.com/microbiome-gut-bacteria-wine-coffee-384151>.

9. 'NEWS: Drinking a Glass of Wine and Taking a Walk May Be Key to Longevity.' Blue Zone, 20 February 2018. <www.bluezones.com/2018/02/drinking-glass-wine-taking-walk-may-be-key-to-longevity/>.

10. McIntyre, Annie. *The Complete Herbal Tutor*. Octopus Publishing Group, Gaia Division: London, 2010.

Chapter 12: The Kefir Solution Step #5: Make Lifestyle Shifts

1. McIntyre, Annie. *The Complete Herbal Tutor*. Octopus Publishing Group, Gaia Division: London. 2010.

2. University of California, Los Angeles, Health Sciences. 'New form of irritable bowel syndrome occurs after patients suffer acute diverticulitis.' ScienceDaily. *ScienceDaily*, 5 September 2013. <www.sciencedaily.com/releases/2013/09/130905160410.htm>.

3. Koutroubakis, I.E. 'Serum laminin and collagen IV in inflammatory bowel disease.' *Journal of Clinical Pathology*. Nov 2003. <www.ncbi.nlm.nih.gov/pubmed/14600124>.

4. Axe, Josh. 'What is Collagen? 7 Ways Collagen Can Boost Your Health.' *Food is Medicine*. <www.draxe.com/what-is-collagen/>.

5. Children's Hospital & Research Center Oakland. 'Causal link found between vitamin D, serotonin synthesis and autism in new study.' ScienceDaily. *ScienceDaily*, 26 February 2014. <www.sciencedaily.com/releases/2014/02/140226110836.htm>.

6. UCSF Benioff Children's Hospital Oakland. 'Omega 3 fatty acids, vitamin D may control brain serotonin, affecting behavior and psychiatric disorders.' ScienceDaily. *ScienceDaily*, 25 February 2015. <www.sciencedaily.com/releases/2015/02/150225094109.htm>.

7. University of Sheffield. 'Large proportion of IBS sufferers are vitamin D deficient.' ScienceDaily. *ScienceDaily*, 21 December 2015. <www.sciencedaily.com/releases/2015/12/151221071924.htm>.

8. Mundasad, Smitha. 'Vitamin D supplements advised for everyone.' BBC News. Health. 21 July 2016. <www.bbc.co.uk/news/health-36846894>.

9. Sublette, M.E. 'Meta-analysis of the effects of eicosapentaenoic acid (EPA) in clinical trials in depression.' *Journal of Clinical Psychiatry.* 6 September 2011. <www.ncbi.nlm.nih.gov/pubmed/21939614>.

10. van der Hulst, R.R.W.J. et al. 'Glutamine and the preservation of gut integrity.' *The Lancet.* Volume 341, No. 8857, p.1363–65, 29 May 1993. <www.thelancet.com/journals/lancet/article/PII0140-6736(93)90939-E/abstract>.

11. Huffman, F.G. 'L-glutamine supplementation improves nelfinavir-associated diarrhea in HIV-infected individuals.' *HIV Clin Trials.* 2003 Sep–Oct;4(5):324–9. <www.ncbi.nlm.nih.gov/pubmed/14583848>.

12. Vanderbilt University Medical Center. 'New Role For Serotonin "Ironed Out".' ScienceDaily. *ScienceDaily*, 29 January 2009. <www.sciencedaily.com/releases/2009/01/090127123009.htm>.

13. University of Michigan Health System. 'Pain In The Gut? Don't Blame Stomach Acid; University Of Michigan Scientists Show Why Inhibiting Acid Production Could Make Gastritis Worse.' ScienceDaily. *ScienceDaily*, 15 January 2002. <www.sciencedaily.com/releases/2002/01/020115074441.htm>.

14. Ibid.

15. Mayo Clinic. 'Proton pump inhibitors decrease diversity in gut microbiome, increase risk for complications.' ScienceDaily. *ScienceDaily*, 25 November 2014. <www.sciencedaily.com/releases/2014/11/141125074656.htm>.

16. Ibid.

17. Mayo Clinic. 'Proton pump inhibitors decrease diversity in gut microbiome, increase risk for complications.' ScienceDaily. *ScienceDaily*, 25 November 2014. <www.sciencedaily.com/releases/2014/11/141125074656.htm>.

18. Ibid.

19. Whiteman, Honor. 'A leisurely walk can boost mood, psychological well-being.' *Medical News Today.* 13 May 2017. <www.medicalnewstoday.com/articles/317451.php?iacp>.

20. Cohut, Maria. 'Just 1 hour of exercise per week could prevent depression.' *Medical News Today*, 3 October 2017. <www.medicalnewstoday.com/articles/319607.php?utm_source=newsletter&utm_medium=email&utm_campaign=weekly>.

21. University of Gothenburg. 'Exercise improve symptoms in irritable bowel syndrome.' ScienceDaily. *ScienceDaily*, 25 January 2011. <www.sciencedaily.com/releases/2011/01/110125092231.htm>.

22. American Gastroenterological Association. 'Physical Inactivity Worsens GI Symptoms In Obese People.' ScienceDaily. *ScienceDaily*, 3 October 2005. <www.sciencedaily.com/releases/2005/10/051003080847.htm>.

23. *Journal of Alternative and Complementary Medicine*, 2017; (doi: 10.1089/acm.2016.0140)

24. University of Bristol. 'Getting Dirty May Lift Your Mood.' ScienceDaily. *ScienceDaily*, 10 April 2007. <www.sciencedaily.com/releases/2007/04/070402102001.htm>.

25. Ibid.

26. University of Illinois College of Agricultural, Consumer and Environmental Sciences. 'Immune system may be pathway between nature and good health.' ScienceDaily. *ScienceDaily*, 16 September 2015. <www.sciencedaily.com/releases/2015/09/150916162120.htm>.

27. Ibid.

28. University of Illinois College of Agricultural, Consumer and Environmental Sciences. 'Immune system may be pathway between nature and good health.' ScienceDaily. *ScienceDaily*, 16 September 2015. <www.sciencedaily.com/releases/2015/09/150916162120.htm>.

29. Ibid.

30. University of Illinois College of Agricultural, Consumer and Environmental Sciences. 'Immune system may be pathway between nature and good health.' ScienceDaily. *ScienceDaily*, 16 September 2015. <www.sciencedaily.com/releases/2015/09/150916162120.htm>.

31. University of Gothenburg. 'Hypnosis should be offered to patients with IBS, Swedish research suggests.' ScienceDaily. *ScienceDaily*, 18 December 2012. <www.sciencedaily.com/releases/2012/12/121218094234.htm>.

32. Vanderbilt University. 'Type of psychotherapy matters in treatment of irritable bowel syndrome.' ScienceDaily. *ScienceDaily*, 12 December 2016. <www.sciencedaily.com/releases/2016/12/161212152705.htm>.

33. Loyola University Health System. 'Health psychologists now treating functional heartburn, Crohn's Disease, IBS and other GI disorders.' ScienceDaily. *ScienceDaily*, 23 March 2017. <www.sciencedaily.com/releases/2017/03/170323141632.htm>.

34. Vanderbilt University. 'Type of psychotherapy matters in treatment of irritable bowel syndrome.' ScienceDaily. *ScienceDaily*, 12 December 2016. <www.sciencedaily.com/releases/2016/12/161212152705.htm>.

35. Axe, Josh. 'Epsom Salt – The Magnesium-Rich, Detoxifying Pain Reliever.' *Food is Medicine*. <https://draxe.com/epsom-salt/>.

36. Ibid.

37. Seelig, M.S. 'Consequences of magnesium deficiency on the enhancement of stress reactions; preventive and therapeutic implications (a review).' *Journal of the American College of Nutrition* 1994 Oct;13(5):429–46.

38. Galland, L. 'Magnesium, stress and neuropsychiatric disorders'. *Magnes Trace Elem*. 1991–1992;10(2–4):287–301.

39. Axe, Josh. 'Epsom Salt – The Magnesium-Rich, Detoxifying Pain Reliever.' *Food is Medicine*. <https://draxe.com/epsom-salt/>.

40. Ibid.

41. Ibid.

42. Ibid..

Further reading and resources

If you want to find out more about the fascinating world of the human microbiome, and learn how to apply natural health principles, I highly recommend reading the work of the following experts:

Dr Josh Axe: *Eat Dirt: Why Leaky Gut May Be the Root Cause of Your Health Problems and 5 Surprising Steps to Cure It*. HarperWave, 2016

Dr Natasha Campbell-McBride: *Gut and Psychology Syndrome: Natural Treatment for Autism, ADD/ADHD, Dyslexia, Dyspraxia, Depression, Schizophrenia*. Medinform Publishing, 2004

Dr Will Cole: *Ketotarian: The (Mostly) Plant-Based Diet to Burn Fat, Boost Your Energy, Crush Your Cravings, and Calm Inflammation*. Avery Publishing Group, 2018

Dr Mark Hyman: *Eat Fat Get Thin: Why the Fat We Eat Is the Key to Sustained Weight Loss and Vibrant Health*. Sapiens Editorial, 2017

Chris Kresser: *The Paleo Cure: Eat Right for Your Genes, Body Type and Personal Health Needs – Prevent and Reverse Disease, Lose Weight*

Effortlessly and Look and Feel Better than Ever. Little, Brown and Company, 2015

Dr Michael Mosley: *The Clever Guts Diet: How to Revolutionise your Body from the Inside Out.* Short Books Ltd, 2017

Resources

Goat's milk kefir can be ordered from www.chucklinggoat.co.uk. It can be delivered anywhere in mainland Europe – unfortunately we are unable to deliver outside mainland Europe. Check the website, as this may change in time.

Shann's medical teas and ashwagandha can also be ordered from www.chucklinggoat.co.uk.

For medical herbs, I recommend G. Baldwin & Co: www.baldwins. co.uk.

Acknowledgements

The more I learn about ecosystems, the more grateful I am to all the people around me. The strength of any ecosystem lies in the number of *connections* between organisms in it. Writing a book is far from a solo endeavour: it takes an entire forest full of contributors!

So my sincere, grateful and heartfelt thanks go to everyone in my particular ecosystem:

Reid Tracy, President and CEO of Hay House, Inc., who believed in me from the beginning, and has been willing to gamble on me yet again. Your quiet, undemanding support and faith have enabled our family and our business to flourish and grow over the years. Deepest gratitude!

Michelle Pilley, Publisher and Managing Director of Hay House UK, who has held the kite string with unending grace as I've loop the looped my idea kite all over the place. And in the end, she helped reel it all back in and made it fly right! Thank you for letting me have yet another go, Michelle.

Debra Wolter, editor extraordinaire, who was brave enough to co-pilot the raft with me over the editing whitewater rapids. Lovely clarity of mind and lucidity; and patient willingness to engage with the fine details. There's no one I'd rather paddle with: thanks for all the great steers and saves!

Julie Oughton for her big picture insight, **Tom Cole** for his social media and video chops; **Jo Burgess and Sian Orrell** for their brilliant marketing expertise; **Leanne Siu Anastasi** for her inspired cover design; and **all the wonderful team at Hay House** for just being extraordinary and walking their talk as a real mind, body and spirit-based organization. I always heave a deep sigh of relief when I walk into those offices and feel the soul reality of the lovely world you've all created there – still don't take it for granted!

Bonnie Nadell, who has been my agent throughout the decades and my rock to depend on. Thank you Bonnie. You're the best.

My adored husband, Rich, who still amazes me after all these years with his wisdom, love, patience and bad jokes. Couldn't have done any of this without you. Wouldn't have wanted to. Never want to. Writing a book draws heavily on everyone's resources – thank you for carrying me on your back through this process, one more time!

My beautiful family: Ceris, George, Elly, Josh, Joli, Benji and little Macsen. You guys are my happy place.

My parents: Don and Ann Nix, who have been there through the years with support and love, setting the standard for living with artistic integrity, creativity and passion.

Index

B

bacteriophages 60–61
bananas 106, 113, 117, 150
Barber, Caroline Debnam 63–4
barley 134
beans/legumes 106, 117, 118,
    157
  black turtle beans 160–61
  cooking dried beans 141
  kidney beans 113, 157, 161
  removing lectins 138–41
  sprouting 138–41
beef 106, 156
  stew 175–7
biodiversity 6, 110–11
  in the microbiome 110–11,
    124, 183, 202
biotin 149
bitters, with apple cider vinegar
    203–4
Blackwell, Annette 143–4
blood glucose/sugar 125–7, 128
  spikes 126, 147
bone broth 196
Bradshaw, Christine xxiii–xxiv
brain
  binding sites for serotonin 25
  decision-making 82–3
  'default network' 14–15
  emotional and logical sides
    82–3
  fight-or-flight response 68,
    208
  gut–brain axis see gut–brain
    axis
  hypothalamic-pituitary-
    adrenal (HPA) axis 36–7,
    68, 69
  neurons see neurons

neurotransmitters see
    neurotransmitters;
    serotonin
  and psychobiotics 35–8
  response to pain 16–17
  and soil bacteria 206–7
  and tryptophan 88
bread 127, 128, 151
  kefir soda bread 153
breakfast 108, 145, 146–50
breathing, deep 205–6
buckwheat 133, 135, 154, 167
burdock root tea 192
Burnet, Philip 36
butyrate 115

C

calcium 132
calendula tea 193
Campbell-McBride, Natasha 108
candida 6
casein
    A1 130–31, 138
    A2 131
cashews 106, 138
cauliflower 107, 113, 157
Cerdigion, A. J. 51–2
chamomile tea 192, 193
chia seeds 146, 147–8, 157
chicken 106, 108, 156, 159–60,
    161–2
  crunchy almond 177–8
  roast 170–71
  soup 171–2
chickpeas 106, 128, 136–7, 157,
    163–4
  chickpea/gram flour 136–7
chicory 54, 117, 183

ABOUT THE AUTHOR

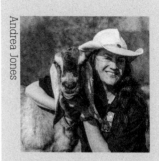

Andrea Jones

Shann Nix Jones was the ultimate American city girl until she fell in love with a Welsh farmer at the age of 41. Shann and her husband, Rich, realized that they could do something extraordinary when they started to work with goats' milk and used it to heal their son's eczema, and Rich's life-threatening superbug infection. They decided to quit their respective day jobs, and try to make a go of the goats'-milk business full time. They now have 70 goats who have become like members of the family.

In April 2011, the couple launched their online business, Chuckling Goat, selling health-enhancing soaps, creams and probiotic kefir drinks, which they make by hand on the farm. The launch was a huge success, and today their award-winning homemade products are available in the United Kingdom and all over the EU.

f chucklinggoat

𝕏 @chucklinggoat

◙ @chucklinggoat

✉ info@chucklinggoat.co.uk

www.chucklinggoat.co.uk

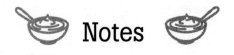

Notes

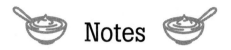# Notes

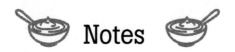

Notes

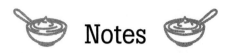

Notes

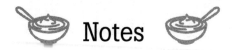 Notes

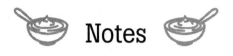

Notes

HAY HOUSE

Look within

Join the conversation about latest products,
events, exclusive offers and more.

f Hay House UK

🐦 @HayHouseUK

📷 @hayhouseuk

💙 healyourlife.com

We'd love to hear from you!